KU-491-899

The Consumer Guide to Mental Health

TRISH GROVES and IAN PENNELL are both doctors who specialized in psychiatry and are members of the Royal College of Psychiatrists.

Trish Groves now works in medical journalism as an assistant editor at the *British Medical Journal*. She also broadcasts on health matters, having presented the DocSpot for TV-a.m. and contributed to radio programmes for the BBC World Service, GLR, and BBC Radio 5. Trish retains a keen interest in psychiatry and recently contributed to and edited a book on the government's community care reforms. She is married and has a son and a daughter.

Ian Pennell is a consultant psychiatrist in the NHS in the West Midlands, treating adults with mental illness. He has a special interest in rehabilitation and community care for people with long-term problems. He has also contributed to a continuing education course for doctors (the *Medicine International* series). Ian is married and has one daughter.

The Consumer Guide to Mental Health

The illnesses, the treatment and
how to get the best out of the help available

Dr Trish Groves & Dr Ian Pennell

HarperCollins*Publishers*

HarperCollins*Publishers*
77–85 Fulham Palace Road,
Hammersmith, London w6 8jb

A Paperback Original 1995

1 3 5 7 9 8 6 4 2

Copyright © Trish Groves and Ian Pennell 1995

The Authors assert the moral right to
be identified as the authors of this work

ISBN 0 00 637590 1

Set in Linotron Palatino by
Rowland Phototypesetting Ltd
Bury St Edmunds, Suffolk

Printed in Great Britain by
HarperCollinsManufacturing Glasgow

Contents

Acknowledgements

The author and the publishers should like to thank the following for their permission to reproduce copyright material:

Marion Boyars for Ken Kesey, *One Flew Over the Cuckoo's Nest*.

BMJ Publishing Group for Moran Campbell, *Not Always on the Level* and P. K. Thomas, 'The Chronic Fatigue Syndrome: What Do We Know?'.

British Journal of Psychiatry for M. A. J. Romme, A. Honig, E. O. Noorthoorn and colleagues, 'Coping with Hearing Voices: An Emancipatory Approach', and for Tyrer P. and colleagues, 'Personality Disorder in Perspective'.

J. M. Dent for Dylan Thomas, *Under Milk Wood*.

Donna Dale Carnegie for Dale Carnegie, *How to Stop Worrying and Start Living*.

Faber & Faber for Elizabeth Forsythe, *Alzheimer's Disease: The Long Bereavement*.

HarperCollins Publishers USA for Thomas S. Szasz, *The Myth of Mental Illness*.

Mrs Laura Huxley and Random House UK Ltd for Aldous Huxley, *Brave New World*.

Independent on Sunday for Angela Neustatter, 'Parental Agony and the Ecstasy'.

Kingsway Publications for Mary Moate and David Enoch, *Schizophrenia: Voices in the Dark*.

Penguin Books for Simone de Beauvoir, *Old Age*, translated by Patrick O'Brian (©Editions Gallimard, translation copyright André Deutsch, Weidenfeld & Nicolson and G. P. Putnam's Sons, 1972.)

Random House for Kingsley Amis, *Jake's Thing*.

Routledge for Pamela Ashurst and Zaida Hall, *Understanding Women in Distress*.

Martin Secker & Warburg Ltd for Colette, *Gigi*.

Sheldon Press for Shirley Trickett, *Coping with Anxiety and Depression*.

The Society of Authors on behalf of the Bernard Shaw Estate for Bernard Shaw, *The Doctor's Dilemma*.

Tavistock Publications for R. D. Laing and A. Esterson, *Sanity, Madness and the Family*.

Introduction

We like to believe that we live in enlightened times and that there is no shame about having a mental illness. However, it is fair to assume that most people would prefer to have a physical illness and go into an ordinary hospital to have medical or surgical treatment than a mental illness and go into a mental hospital under the care of a psychiatrist. Age-old prejudice takes a long time to change. Many sorts of mental illness are now treatable but even these still have some stigma attached . . . Fear about mental illness can be an additional reason that stops the carer asking for help.

From *Alzheimer's Disease: The Long Bereavement* by Elizabeth Forsythe[1]

We both felt as Philip's parents we should be told exactly what was wrong. John decided to ask one of the doctors outright. We realized, of course, that by asking a direct question, we must be prepared for a direct answer. It wasn't at all easy, but we had to know what was wrong. This, we felt, was our right.

When John approached the doctor our worst fears were confirmed. Back came the answer that, yes, in their opinion Philip was suffering from schizophrenia. The doctor was more helpful this time, adding what seemed at the time to be a strange remark! He said that they did not like to use the word 'schizophrenia'. Why not? we wondered. Why the mystery?

From *Schizophrenia: Voices in the Dark* by Mary Moate and David Enoch[2]

WHAT THIS BOOK OFFERS

About half a million people in Britain suffer from schizophrenia: it is three times commoner than cancer. And at any one time up to a tenth of the adult population is ill with depression. But experts are still quite ignorant about the causes and mechanisms of mental illness. No one has really explained how the mass of biological circuitry in the brain can contain the mind, the soul and the personality; let alone how it can all go wrong.

But, even if the experts do not have the answers to the most fundamental questions about mental illness, they have plenty of practical knowledge about probable causes and about relieving symptoms and suffering. Unfortunately, they are not always very good at sharing that knowledge. This is why psychiatry, the medical speciality that diagnoses and treats mental illness, is still surrounded by a certain mystique. And poor understanding of mental illness is the main cause of the prejudice that produces derogatory labels like madman, nutter and loony.

We hope that this book on psychiatry written by two psychiatrists (doctors who have specialized in helping people with mental illnesses) might help to reduce some of this misunderstanding. This is not primarily a guide on self-help or on keeping mentally well. Rather, it is a consumer's guide for adults who use psychiatric services and for their friends and relatives.

This guide is arranged in nine chapters, eight of which are based around types of mental illness that affect adults. Chapter 1 covers stress-related problems including anxiety states, phobias and sexual and relationship problems. Chapter 2 covers depression and manic depression and looks at kinds of depression that particularly affect women. Chapter 3 explains the known facts about schizophrenia while Chapter 4 covers the mental health problem that may eventually affect one in five of us: dementia. In Chapter 5 drug problems are considered, including those arising from use of two socially acceptable drugs: alcohol and nicotine. Anorexia, bulimia nervosa and compulsive eating, common problems or disorders of eating, are looked at in Chapter 6. And Chapter 7 explores a group of problems that psychiatrists regularly diagnose and try to grapple with but the public rarely hears about – the personality disorders. Chapter 8 looks at suicide and parasuicide. Finally, Chapter 9 looks at the ethical and legal problems that arise in psychiatry. And at the end of the book there is a glossary explaining psychiatric jargon and a directory of addresses for voluntary organizations.

These chapters can be used as separate reference sources by people wanting to know about the particular problems affecting them or those close to them. And the whole guide, read through in order, gives a comprehensive view of the medical speciality called psychiatry. In essence it explains what is known about mental illness, what psychiatrists and other mental health professionals do, what happens to people admitted to hospital or offered community care, and what treatment and other support is available through Britain's health and social services. Importantly, this book also acknowledges the vital role of voluntary organizations in advising and supporting people with mental illness.

Overall, this guide is written from a medical viewpoint. We believe that mental illness is as real as a broken leg and that physical treatments like drugs are often necessary. We also believe that much mental illness is as difficult as physical illness to avoid and is not simply a consequence of unhealthy lifestyle or failure to pull yourself together.

In describing the different kinds of mental illness we have used the terms that doctors use. These labels may seem very arbitrary at times. Indeed, experts around the world still disagree over the way in which mental illnesses should be defined and classified. And a few, like the American psychiatrist Thomas S. Szasz, say that mental illness does not even exist and that psychiatric treatment is a purely social action like the work of the police. In his book *The Myth of Mental Illness* Dr Szasz says:

> In psychiatric circles it is almost indelicate to ask: What is mental illness? In non-psychiatric circles mental illness all too often is considered to be whatever psychiatrists say it is. The answer to the question, Who is mentally ill? thus becomes: Those who are confined in mental hospitals or who consult psychiatrists . . .[3]

But intellectual arguments about the existence of mental illness, and whether psychiatry is a medical science, are not very practical and do little to help the many people who suffer from what is – regardless of philosophizing – generally seen as mental illness.

Agreeing with the idea of labels is not necessary to get psychiatric help, but understanding psychiatric jargon should make consultations seem less daunting and concepts of mental health and illness seem a little clearer. Non-medical terms are often even more confusing, after all. One of the commonest – nervous breakdown – is used to cover the first attack of anything from agoraphobia to schizophrenia. All that nervous breakdown means is that the affected person develops a mental health problem which interrupts his or her life for a while. It says nothing about the nature of the problem or its severity and duration. Psychiatrists and other doctors do not talk in terms of nervous breakdowns; they prefer to use more specific and meaningful concepts.

Understanding how psychiatry works helps people who have to use mental health services. For a start, accurate information enables service users to communicate with mental health professionals, some of whom seem to barge in and take complete control, while others seem to stand on the sidelines and do too little. Well-informed patients usually feel confident about putting questions to their doctors and, if necessary, complaining about their care. Secondly, people who know which factors might cause and worsen mental illness can try to prevent it. Thirdly, knowledge about services allows the people who use them to realize that they have choices – they can make informed decisions about the help offered. And they can campaign for a full range of services in their local area if they know what is missing. This is particularly the case for minority groups, for example some ethnic groups who find that existing health services do not recognize or respond to cultural differences in expressing and treating mental illness. In these and other ways, detailed knowledge about mental health problems and their treatment can give sufferers more say and more clout.

Relatives and friends of sufferers also need information about mental illness if they are to understand what is happening and to help. Because a confidential, trusting relationship between a patient and a doctor is central to all medical practice, relatives and other carers are often left in the dark about patients' diagnoses and treatments. This can leave those carers feeling isolated, helpless, and even guilty – particularly if they are told that their responses to certain situations are undermining treatment. Others may feel that they are suspected of doing too little to help. Sometimes relatives and friends just can't win. Better information may help them not to feel this way.

WHAT PSYCHIATRY OFFERS

Psychiatry has to deal with a huge range of patients, including some who seem unhappy with their lives rather than ill, some who seem extremely ill but do not feel it, and some who cannot even communicate. Thus, psychiatry must offer a wide range of treatment approaches.

But before psychiatrists offer treatment they make diagnoses. Psychiatrists have learnt by personal trial and error and collective scientific research that certain signs and symptoms occur in clusters, and that each cluster or syndrome tends to respond to a certain kind of treatment. For example, many people cope with feeling down but those who feel down and have insomnia, tiredness, poor concentration and poor appetite feel ill – clinically depressed – and less able to cope. These additional symptoms usually respond well to antidepressant treatments, confirming in a roundabout way that the diagnosis of depression was correct. The idea that illnesses and syndromes can be diagnosed in this seemingly unscientific way is supported by the fact that symptoms hardly vary among very different sufferers. For instance, a woman of 30 with depression will probably have the same symptoms as a depressed man of 50, and respond to the same treatment. The patients may be very different people, but their depressive illnesses have much in common.

None the less, psychiatrists sometimes find diagnosis very difficult and occasionally have to change their minds about what is wrong. This is partly explained by the long timescale of some illnesses and the gradual, vague way in which they develop. It is fairly common for someone with schizophrenia to attract three or four increasingly serious diagnoses over several years until the illness really shows itself. The other reason why psychiatrists sometimes seem to dither about diagnosis is that they try to err on the side of caution and avoid labelling illnesses (and, indirectly, people) until the picture is really clear. Therefore a psychiatrist might not immediately diagnose schizophrenia in a patient with only one or two of the many symptoms that characterize it. Helping the few symptoms and waiting to see whether they clear up or worsen before deciding on a diagnosis is sometimes the most reasonable approach.

Although uncertainties like these are important to understand, they arise relatively rarely. Most mental health problems can be diagnosed and treated by general practitioners and their teams without being referred for specialist psychiatric help. And another direct source of help, the community mental health centre, is becoming increasingly available.

Direct Sources of Medical Help for Mental Health Problems
The main providers of mental health care are general practitioners, not psychiatrists. According to government figures, GPs treat nine out of ten recognized mental health problems and see some 12 million adults with symptoms of mental illness each year. Even for the one in ten of these patients referred to psychiatrists, GPs should be told enough about

the diagnosis and treatment to know how to help with problems that continue or recur.

To make this feedback process smoother and to make referral less daunting, as many as one in five psychiatrists now see patients at their doctors' surgeries. Psychiatric nurses, social workers, psychologists, counsellors and therapists now work on a sessional basis at many local surgeries. And if assessment at the surgery or health centre is impractical or inappropriate for some reason, each of these specialists can do home visits.

Community mental health centres also offer a short cut to psychiatric help. The idea for these centres came from the United States, where those who cannot afford to pick up the phone book and choose a private psychiatrist under health insurance can go to local state-run mental health centres for psychiatric help. The centres are like general practice health centres but they cater solely for mental health problems, offering assessment and practical help five days a week during office hours. Typically, these centres have a staff of eight to ten – nurses, therapists, social workers and psychiatrists – and offer support groups, relaxation classes, and art therapy, among many services. Most new attenders are referred by their GPs, but some centres run open access sessions when people with problems can arrange their own appointments or even turn up unannounced. Community mental health centres have opened gradually in Britain since the 1980s and are not available in all areas. And not all are staffed by psychiatrists. The more traditional, and still more common, route to a psychiatrist is from the GP to a hospital outpatient department.

Specialist Psychiatric Help

Psychiatric help is provided by many professionals with different training backgrounds and roles: psychiatrists, psychologists, nurses, occupational therapists, psychotherapists and social workers all play a part.

A psychiatrist is a fully trained doctor who specializes in diagnosing and treating people with mental health problems.

Basic training for all doctors (see Box 1) comprises two years at university, studying human life sciences such as anatomy, physiology and biochemistry. This is followed by three years spent learning medical practice in hospital wards and clinics, culminating in the final exams that transform the students into doctors. After five years at medical school, doctors work a probationary year as junior house officers before their names can be entered in the medical register. Then they can pick one branch of medicine but must continue to train as they work and must pass postgraduate exams before they can be considered specialists.

Strictly speaking, the term psychiatrist should be applied only to a consultant. But, in common with most branches of medicine, psychiatry gives its trainees plenty of clinical experience and relies on them to share much of the workload. Many doctors working on psychiatric wards and in outpatient clinics are senior house officers and registrars. They have learnt the skills required to assess patients but are supervised by consultants in making diagnoses and deciding on any treatment.

BOX 1	*Medical training*	

	Medical school: 5 years
	    FINALS
	Junior house officer: 1 year
	    SPECIALIZATION
	Senior house officer: 1–3 years
		} MEDICAL STUDENT

	Registrar: 2–3 years SPECIALIST EXAMS Senior registrar: 3–4 years Consultant: 20–30 years	} DOCTOR

Assessment and Diagnosis

In many ways a visit to a psychiatrist is much like any trip to a hospital doctor. Indeed, psychiatric clinics are often based in the outpatient departments of general hospitals. But, unusually, first appointments with psychiatrists can last an hour or more because the psychiatrist, and sometimes other members of the team like nurses, doctors in training and social workers, need to ask lots of questions and record the whole consultation in a set of confidential case notes.

Explaining personal problems to more than one person might seem difficult, but teamwork is often the best approach in psychiatry, and it is worth sticking with. Being ill is often a joint effort too, involving and affecting close relatives and friends, so patients are frequently asked to bring a relative or friend to be interviewed at the same time in another room.

Psychiatric assessment follows a pretty standard format that includes an interview and an examination and is sometimes backed up by a range of tests.

THE PSYCHIATRIC INTERVIEW

The interview starts with the patient's history. The history is just what it sounds like – a personal story that explains how and, to some extent, why help is needed now. A doctor assessing someone wanting help for varicose veins would ask for details of their physical health and lifestyle (Do you have to stand up all day at work? Do other members of your family have varicose veins?) to make a decision about treatment and likely outcome. Mental health problems almost invariably develop from a mixture of causes – emotional, social, physical and familial – and it helps psychiatrists to know what the people they see are normally like and what kind of lives they have led (see Boxes 2–5 for details of the questions psychiatrists ask routinely). These questions may seem unnecessarily intrusive, but they allow psychiatrists to understand patients' problems and decide on the best way to help them.

The next stage in assessment is the mental state examination. This is how psychiatrists examine minds, or at least their current state. Mental state examination is not as difficult as it sounds. It entails more questions and careful observation to assess feelings and thoughts and how well the mind is working (for example, in terms of memory and concentration). We all give off clues about the way we feel –

psychiatrists are simply trained to tune in to them. For example, a severely depressed person may look sad and unanimated and a bit dishevelled and may find concentration hard, expressing gloomy ideas in a slow monotone. It may take gentle but thorough questioning to establish the extent to which that depression has taken hold.

During the mental state examination the psychiatrist is only doing what we all do when we meet people – forming an impression of both personality and current state of mind. The difference between this consultation and a social interaction is that the psychiatrist is trained to ask specific personal questions, listen closely to the answers, and observe body language. The mental state examination does not involve psychoanalysis or mind-reading. It is simply the way that psychiatrists look for signs and symptoms of mental illness.

It is not surprising that, with all this information being gathered, the first meeting with a psychiatrist takes at least an hour. Contrary to popular belief, patients seeing psychiatrists do not lie on couches unless they need physical check-ups. During first consultations psychiatrists usually make diagnoses and explain them. Of course, there may not always be a diagnosis to make. The boundary between a life problem that will clear up spontaneously and a mental illness that needs treatment is sometimes quite blurred. GPs occasionally have to refer patients to psychiatrists to be on the safe side. In a situation like this, one long talk with a psychiatrist may be enough to put the problem in perspective and help the person to sort it out without professional help.

Sometimes more information is needed to make a firm diagnosis or assess the full extent of a problem. Further assessment in the clinic may be necessary, or some additional tests. Simple blood tests can be done in outpatient clinics but other investigations will mean referral to a different department, usually on another day.

BOX 2

> **The full psychiatric history I**
> *Medical and psychiatric history*
>
> Who made the referral to the psychiatric team?
>
> Why now?
>
> What is the problem?
>
> When did the problem start?
>
> How did the problem start and how has it developed?
>
> How has the problem affected your life?
>
> Have you had psychological problems in the past? Describe in detail – symptoms and diagnosis (if made), type and source of any treatment, outcome.
>
> Have you had physical illnesses? Describe in detail, as above.
>
> Are you taking any medicines? Give details of names, doses, duration.
>
> Have you had bad reactions to any medicines or treatments?
>
> How much do you drink/smoke?
>
> Have you ever used illegal drugs? Give details.

BOX 3

> **Psychiatric history II**
> *Family history: details of parents and all siblings*
>
> Ages of family members.
>
> If dead – at what age? How? How old were you at the time?
>
> Occupation.

Marital status.

Personality.

Relationship with you.

Health. If poor, give details.

Did/does anyone in the family have
psychiatric problems?

BOX 4

Psychiatric history III

Personal history

CHILDHOOD
When and where were you born?

Were there any physical problems around
birth and in childhood?

At what ages did you start and leave school?

How did you get on at school (with friends,
teachers, work)?

What kind of teenager were you?

What qualifications did you attain?

OCCUPATION
At what age did you start work?

What jobs have you held?

Have you had any problems at work?

RELATIONSHIPS AND SEX
When did puberty start?

Have you had past or present problems with
your sex life?

What close relationships have you had?

Are you married? If so, for how long?

How old is your partner, and what job does he or she do?

Are you having relationship problems now?

Do you have any children? (Have any died, been miscarried or aborted?)

How old, and how healthy are they?

How do you get on with them?

BOX 5

Psychiatric history IV

Social life and problems

Do you have any problems with finance or housing?

Who are your main supports?

How do you get on with your friends?

Have you been in trouble with the law?

Personality

What sort of person are you?

What is your mood most of the time?

What do you think of yourself and what you have done in life?

How do you enjoy yourself and spend your spare time?

Do you have strong religious or moral beliefs?

Do you have any habits that bother you?

FURTHER ASSESSMENT AND TESTS

Psychological tests These will be performed by a clinical psychologist, a non-medical specialist who has a degree in psychology and has had postgraduate training to acquire detailed knowledge of the thought and behaviour patterns of people with mental health problems. Psychologists work within or alongside the psychiatric team, helping in both assessment and treatment. The range of psychological tests study memory, intelligence, personality, perception, and capability for abstract thinking. Most tests entail questionnaires or puzzles, rather like those personality quizzes in magazines that ask 'If you were in a certain situation and a certain event occurred, would you (i) . . . (ii) . . . or (iii) . . . ?' and then tell you that you are lovable, bossy, or whatever. Similar tests are used in education and industry to test aptitude and ability.

Physical tests   Although researchers have identified small physical abnormalities in the brains of some people with mental illnesses, the meaning of these findings is not yet clear. And there is little evidence that routine physical investigation is useful in diagnosing psychiatric illnesses. However, tests may be important in ruling out physical illnesses that can cause psychological symptoms and masquerade as psychiatric illnesses. The physical tests used in psychiatry are summarized in Box 6. If you are advised to have any of them, they will be explained to you by the staff in the departments where they are performed.

BOX 6   **Physical tests used in psychiatry**

Blood tests – for anaemia, metabolic disturbance, infection

Skull X-ray – for fractures and other structural abnormalities

Brain imaging

- electroencephalography (abbreviated to EEG): tracing the electric signals or waves that the brain generates

- angiography: X-rays using dye to show blood vessels

- computed tomography (abbreviated to CT or CAT scanning): X-rays guided by computer to give pictures in 'slices'

- single photon emission computed tomography (abbreviated to SPECT): a recent variant of CT scanning

- nuclear magnetic resonance (abbreviated to NMR): using strong magnetic fields to make the nuclei of hydrogen atoms in the body spin and give off radio waves that are scanned and built into a picture

- positron emission tomography (abbreviated to PET scanning): the patient is given a minute dose of a radioactive substance that combines with particular brain chemicals and gives off subatomic particles called positrons. These and, therefore, the site of the brain chemicals being studied, are detected by the scanner.

Social assessment Many patients have social difficulties that can be teased out and helped by a psychiatric social worker. Psychiatric social workers train at university or college to understand all aspects of social and mental welfare. They know about financial, domestic, and housing difficulties as well as legal rights. 'Approved social workers' have special training in the use of the Mental Health Act, the law that authorizes compulsory admissions to hospital and compulsory psychiatric treatments. These social workers also know about all the mental health services offered by local councils and voluntary organizations and can refer clients to them. The role of some social workers has been enlarged in recent years by the expansion of community care (see p. xxxvi).

Occupational therapy assessment Mental health problems causing practical disabilities – for instance, inability to work because of depression, agitation and poor concentration – can be assessed and helped by occupational therapists. Occupational therapists are trained and qualified at college to help sufferers regain self-confidence, independence, and practical skills like shopping and cooking.

Treatment

The aim of psychiatric treatment is to help sufferers shake off, or at least cope with, symptoms and to gain or regain an acceptable quality of life. Sometimes treatment merely speeds up recovery that would occur spontaneously, but may be justified because it reduces the duration and degree of suffering experienced.

Treatment includes psychological, physical, social and occupational components that reflect the wide-reaching effects of mental illness. A general description of these treatments follows: more details will be given later.

PSYCHOLOGICAL TREATMENT

Counselling Counselling is a widely used 'talking cure', particularly in general practice. Counsellors listen to their clients, help them to explore feelings, and to find personal and practical solutions to their problems. Counsellors do not probe into clients' pasts or analyse them, and do not give out advice.

Since the 1970s increasing numbers of GPs have employed trained counsellors to work in their surgeries and health centres. Research suggests that counselling for people with mental health problems reduces the number of consultations with and prescriptions from GPs.

Where counselling is not available through a general practice health centre, trained and supervised private counsellors can be recommended by the British Association of Counselling, whose address is given in Appendix 2. There are also many specialist counselling associations such as Relate, which helps people with relationship problems and was previously known as the Marriage Guidance Council.

Psychotherapy This is the best known 'talking cure'. Psychotherapy is available on the NHS for individuals, groups and families, but is relatively scarce and oversubscribed, and there may be a wait of many months before starting to see a therapist.

The term psychotherapy is a generalization covering many different concepts. They all started, however, with Sigmund Freud, the father of modern psychotherapy. Freud was a doctor who, along with a number of other researchers in the early 20th century, tried to unravel the mysteries of human mental functioning. He discovered that, as well as the conscious thoughts that guide our feelings and actions, there are powerful psychological forces of which we are not usually aware. Freud proposed a model of the mind with several distinct parts, including sources of unconscious thoughts and primitive instincts. Applying his theories to his patients' freely expressed thoughts, Freud was able to cure many illnesses, some of which had been presumed completely physical. This was the beginning of individual analytical psychotherapy, or psychoanalysis.

Although Freud's principles underpin all subsequent theories about the psyche, many different schools of thought (sometimes contradicting each other) have emerged and influenced psychotherapists. The theoretical differences are beyond the scope of this book, but we recommend below other sources of information for those readers interested to know more. Regardless of the theoretical schools to which various psychotherapists profess allegiance, certain common features apply to all forms of psychotherapy.

Firstly, clients are assessed to see if their personality and their problems are suitable for psychotherapy. Research has shown that this kind of treatment is unlikely to work for certain patients (mainly those who are completely unable to talk about or get in touch with their emotions, those with serious mental illnesses called psychoses, and those with serious dependence on drugs or alcohol). Secondly, clients have to make therapeutic contracts with their therapists, agreeing at the start on the number and timing of therapy sessions and on the outcomes that they hope to achieve. Lastly, the strength of these contracts and the freedom of emotional expression allows clients to develop special (albeit temporary) relationships with their therapists.

Dr Anthony Storr, a consultant psychotherapist, calls psychotherapy 'the art of alleviating personal difficulties through the agency of words and a personal, professional relationship.' As Dr Storr explains in his book *The Art of*

Psychotherapy,[4] the success of psychotherapy probably depends more on these common factors than on the type of analysis. He believes that the marked differences between analytic schools will soon disappear and that the labels 'Freudian', 'Jungian' and 'Kleinian' will become less important. Dr Storr maintains that one or two psychotherapy sessions a week (the most that the NHS is likely to offer, even though some theorists insist on daily therapy) can be very valuable for many patients.

Much NHS psychotherapy is provided by psychiatrists, nurses, social workers, psychologists, and occupational therapists. They are supervised regularly by fully trained psychotherapists (usually consultant psychiatrists who have specialized in psychotherapy), with whom they discuss patients' progress and from whom they get advice. The Royal College of Psychiatrists insists that all doctors training in psychiatry must obtain supervised experience in psychotherapy before sitting their final specialist exams. Some psychotherapists are worried by this. Derek Gale is a non-medical therapist who believes that the NHS psychotherapy service's reliance on such unspecialized staff militates against adequate psychotherapy. In *What is Psychotherapy?*[5] he argues that doctors, in particular, have superior attitudes to and poor understanding of psychotherapy. The other side of the coin, of course, is that patients can at least be reassured that NHS therapists have some related training, that no money has changed hands, and that, should anything go wrong, worsening mental illness can be spotted early on.

Another critic of psychotherapy, Dr Gavin Andrews from Sydney, Australia, says that the treatment does not work and can even be harmful. In an article in the *British Journal of Psychiatry* in 1993, Dr Andrews reviewed research studies and showed that psychotherapy is more expensive and less effective than behaviour therapy (see below) or good general psychiatric care.[6] Harm may arise from two aspects of psychotherapy, said Dr Andrews. Firstly, intense soul-searching prompted by inexperienced therapists can demoralize clients and inhibit recovery. Secondly, the intimate and important relationship that occurs during therapy allows a few psychotherapists to exert undue and unethical influence over clients' lives, even going so far as to have sexual relationships with them. Psychotherapy's advocates have fought back against Dr Andrews, however, saying that the research he cited was not sophisticated enough to show real benefits from psychotherapy and that his arguments about cost are based on Australian health care, in which long-term psychotherapy is used much more widely than in the UK.[7]

Whatever the rights and wrongs of providing psychotherapy, many patients who do want it have little choice of therapist in the UK. If Anthony Storr is right, those patients who cannot afford private psychotherapy and are lucky enough to be offered one of the scarce NHS slots should take up the opportunity with reasonable confidence. For an excellent guide to psychotherapy's many variations and controversies, try the books listed in Box 7.

BOX 7 | **Further reading on psychotherapy**
Talking to a Stranger: a Consumer's Guide to Therapy by Lindsay Knight (Fontana/Collins, 1986). This excellent book explains the different theoretical schools and gives practical advice on how to find and use a trained private therapist.

One to One: Experiences of Psychotherapy by Rosemary Dinnage (Penguin Books, London, 1989). A fascinating and readable collection of personal histories of people who have had psychotherapy.

Against Therapy by Jeffrey Masson (Fontana Paperbacks, London, 1990). A highly controversial critique of modern psychotherapy by a psychoanalyst who believes that we need more kindly friends and fewer professionals.

Behaviour therapy   This is rather more an 'action cure' than a 'talking cure'. Behaviour therapy springs from psychological theories on human behaviour, many of which are based on studies of animals. The therapists, usually clinical psychologists, help people through looking at problematic behaviour patterns and changing them. Behaviour therapists do not generally attempt to uncover anything about clients' pasts or innermost feelings, although one technique called cognitive behaviour therapy looks at current problems in the context of past experiences and thinking patterns. The range of behaviour therapies is shown in Box 8.

BOX 8   **Behaviour therapies**

Relaxation

- The patient is taught to recognize the signs of muscular tension and is shown how to abolish them by a series of exercises.

Exposure therapy

- Systematic desensitization – the anxious patient is gradually exposed to the anxiety-provoking stimulus and taught how to cope with it by relaxation.

- Flooding – the patient is exposed to the stimulus all in one go, with support.

Modelling

- The therapist plays a role to show the patient how to behave, then gives support and feedback to the patient who copies the same action.

Cognitive therapy

- The therapist shows the patient that ways of thinking when ill (particularly pessimism and nihilism when depressed) may lead to misleading interpretations of the world and may influence emotions and psychological symptoms. The therapist teaches positive thinking.

PHYSICAL TREATMENTS

The most widely used physical treatments in psychiatry are drugs. Because the most commonly used drugs will be described in detail in the clinical sections of this book, only a broad summary will be given here. There are a huge number of drugs, and many of them differ only slightly from others in the same category. Many hospitals and general practices make sense of this oversupply by limiting doctors to an agreed list of drugs that includes a reasonable choice from each category.

Hypnotics and sedatives like nitrazepam (trade name Mogadon) calm nerves and cause sleepiness and can be used to treat insomnia. But most insomnia can be treated without drugs and even when a drug is needed, an antidepressant is often better because much insomnia is actually due to depression. Doctors are strongly discouraged from prescribing tranquillizing and anxiety-reducing drugs like diazepam (or Valium) because these drugs are addictive. They are now recommended only for short-term relief of anxiety that is severe, disabling, or unacceptably distressing, or for short-term treatment during drying out from alcohol.

Antidepressants like amitriptyline (Tryptizol, Lentizol) and fluoxetine (Prozac) are given to lift a depressed person's mood and to relieve the physical symptoms that sometimes occur in depression, such as insomnia and poor appetite. Antidepressants' side effects are mostly relatively mild, although one group can lead to sudden and dangerous high blood pressure if taken with certain foods.

Depression is not the only kind of mood problem that may need drug treatment: its opposite extreme, mania, and the mixed problem manic depression virtually always have to be treated with mood-stabilizing drugs. Lithium (Priadel, Camcolit) is used in acute mania to normalize (or stabilize) mood and get rid of the associated psychotic symptoms, hallucinations and delusions. It can also be used in acute depression. However, lithium's main use is to prevent relapse in manic depression. Long-term unwanted effects may include kidney and thyroid problems. Short-term neurological and kidney problems may occur if the blood concentration of lithium is too high – therefore it must be monitored by regular blood tests. Carbamazepine (Tegretol) is a treatment for epilepsy which has been found to stabilize mood. It also necessitates blood tests.

Antipsychotic drugs, also called neuroleptics and major tranquillizers, are the only effective treatments for relieving serious mental illnesses with hallucinations and delusions. They are used mainly in schizophrenia and they include the short-acting drugs chlorpromazine (Largactil) and clozapine (Clozaril) and the long-lasting injections given once every few weeks like fluphenazine decanoate (Modecate). In the long term, however, most antipsychotic drugs can cause a brain problem called tardive dyskinesia that affects control of movement and is not always reversible. And, unwieldy though it may seem, the antipsychotic drugs' short-term side effects such as shaking and stiffness sometimes have to be counteracted by other drugs called anticholinergic drugs. Procyclidine (Kemadrin) and benzhexol (Artane) are commonly used anticholinergic drugs.

The other two physical treatments used in psychiatry are particularly controversial: electroconvulsive therapy (ECT) and psychosurgery. In ECT, which is used mainly to treat severe life-threatening depression, a small electric current is passed through the brain to induce a fit or seizure. Before the treatment the patient is anaesthetized and given a muscle-relaxing injection that reduces the fit to a slight twitching or shaking. Psychosurgery – operating on the brain to alleviate psychiatric illness or difficult personality traits – is extremely uncommon these days. It was once practised widely in Britain but is now performed in only one or two hospitals on highly selected patients with intractable problems. Stereotactic surgery, in which small cuts are made in specific brain fibres under X-ray guidance, has superseded the more generalized lobotomies of old. The important point to make here about this highly specialized treatment is that there are strong legal safeguards against its misuse. The Mental Health Act 1983 ensures that psychosurgery is performed only when the patient has given fully informed consent and a second opinion has agreed that it is necessary. For all other psychiatric treatments (except another rare treatment, hormone implantation for reducing the sex drive of sex offenders) either consent or a second opinion is needed, not both.

OTHER FORMS OF TREATMENT AND HELP

Being mentally ill can reduce sufferers' abilities to cope with many facets of normal life. People who lose the confidence or concentration needed to cook, shop, and budget, or even just socialize can get help from occupational therapists. Art therapy can help the healing process too, allowing expression of feelings that might be difficult to put into words.

Settings for Treatment

Whenever possible, people with mental health problems are seen as outpatients – at home, in their doctors' surgeries, or at psychiatry clinics. People needing specialized or intensive treatment can use a wide range of psychiatric facilities according to their age and special needs (see Box 9). This book is about psychiatric help for adults with mental health problems. It does not, therefore, cover services for children and for people with learning disabilities (mental handicaps). These groups have quite different needs and have their own separate services. Services for children with emotional and behavioural problems are run by a mixture of disciplines – education, social services, psychology and psychiatry. Children and teenagers with psychological problems may be referred by their teachers, social workers, school doctors and nurses, or GPs for help. The first port of call is usually a child-guidance clinic.

People with learning disabilities (low IQ or mental handicap) were, until about 20 years ago, usually cared for in large, rural long-stay hospitals. More recently it has become clear that institutional care is not only unnecessary, but is also detrimental to most people with these problems. Many live at home with their families, or in small residential units that are much homelier than the old hospitals and make work and leisure in ordinary community life much more accessible. Some people with learning disabilities, however, also have mental illnesses. Most can be treated as outpatients, but a few need more intensive inpatient treatment, and a very small minority with disturbed behaviour need secure (i.e. locked) settings.

BOX 9

Specialized facilities offered by psychiatry for different groups

Adults aged 18–70

Community mental health resource centres, outpatient clinics, day hospitals

Admission wards for acute illness

Mother-and-baby units for postnatal illnesses

Long-stay and rehabilitation wards for chronic illness

Alcohol and drug abuse units

Psychotherapy units, e.g. therapeutic communities for daily group therapy

Community care residential units, e.g. hostels, group homes

Elderly people

Day units

Admission/assessment wards

Respite care wards for patients whose relatives need short breaks from caring for them

Long-stay wards, particularly for people with senile dementia

Mentally disturbed offenders

Locked wards

Regional secure units

Special hospitals, e.g. Broadmoor, Rampton

Prison psychiatric units

Children and adolescents

Child-guidance clinics

Day units

Inpatient units

People with learning disabilities (mental handicaps)

Residential hostels

Day centres and hospitals

Inpatient hospitals

TREATING PSYCHIATRIC EMERGENCIES

Psychiatric emergencies may develop from psychological, physical, or practical crises. A psychological crisis (for example after a sudden bereavement) is usually experienced as severe acute distress and inability to cope any longer without help. A physical crisis may develop if a psychological problem causes self-neglect (for example failure to eat) or self-harm (intoxication by alcohol or drugs, self-mutilation, attempted suicide). A practical crisis may occur when personal circumstances change (marital separation, eviction), or when someone's behaviour disturbs other people so much that they cannot cope. Any of these crises may need quick professional intervention.

Relatives and friends often have to get this urgent help. Firstly, they should ring the disturbed or distressed person's GP. If the GP is not available and help is needed very urgently, relatives or friends should phone the local social services department and ask for the duty social worker (on 24-hour call). In a dire emergency, when neither of the first two options are practical, the police will know what to do.

Sometimes the need for intervention is so urgent that admission to hospital will go ahead even if a patient refuses it. Any disturbed adult who threatens his or her own or others' health and safety, and refuses psychiatric help, may be moved and detained by law. The Mental Health Act of 1983 authorizes emergency assessment and treatment of any person with apparent psychiatric problems that fulfil these criteria. This is explained in detail in Chapter 9.

Although admission to hospital may be the best solution, there are other ways that psychiatry can respond to emergencies. In some districts there are 'crisis intervention' teams of psychiatrists, nurses, and social workers who can visit patients urgently at home (at a GP's request) and, sometimes, avert unnecessary admission. And some researchers have shown that home treatment for a range of acute psychiatric problems can be effective.[8]

BOX 10	**How to get urgent psychiatric help for a disturbed relative or friend – 24 hours a day**
	Ring the person's family doctor
	If the doctor can't come quickly, ring the local social services department and ask for the duty social worker
	Failing any response, call the police

TREATMENT IN HOSPITAL

Soon after arriving in hospital new patients are interviewed at least twice. Firstly, a nurse shows the new patient round the ward and takes a brief history. Then the ward doctor will embark on a fully detailed history and examination, including a physical check-up and some blood tests. These interviews will take place in private. On admission, or at a later date, both nursing and medical staff may want to speak to patients' relatives or friends too.

Psychiatric wards do not look like medical or surgical wards and staff may not wear uniforms. Patients do not need to be in their beds during the day, so the beds are situated in separate dormitories. The main part of most wards is a living space with a day room, an activity and television room, quiet rooms, a dining room, and a kitchen. Tea, coffee and meals are usually self-served from trolleys delivered to the ward. Patients may be expected to take turns in helping to serve meals, on a rota basis.

Ward life usually has a certain routine. The day often starts with a community meeting at which patients and nurses discuss issues that affect the whole ward. Patients may go to the occupational therapy department during the day, but there may be also be some therapy groups on the ward, such as relaxation classes.

Doctors do not usually spend all day on the ward. They share their time between several wards, outpatient clinics, and community units. But they do come to the ward at certain fixed times, particularly for ward rounds. In medical and surgical wards, the consultant and his team of doctors and nurses walk from bed to bed, seeing each patient. This is practical for the staff, and for bed-bound patients, but does not allow for private discussion: the whole ward can listen. Psychiatric ward rounds do not go round at all; they take place in conference rooms into which patients can be invited one at a time to see the team. This has the advantage of privacy, but it can be daunting to walk into a room full of people who have just been discussing you. Nevertheless, this is a chance to meet the whole team and ask them questions.

Patients' symptoms and problems are assessed continuously during a stay in hospital. When patients seem well enough they are allowed home for trial periods; initially for one day, then for a night, then for a weekend. If trial leave goes well, discharge can be arranged. Patients are usually asked to attend the outpatient clinic for at least one check-up after a few weeks.

LONG-TERM TREATMENT AND COMMUNITY CARE
Long-term treatment can often be provided by GPs with support and guidance from outpatient psychiatric services. That

is fine for people whose problems allow them to look after themselves and for those with plenty of support from family and friends.

But some people need much more intensive long-term treatment. And many need help with daily life including shopping and cooking, finance, and accommodation. In the past, patients with this degree of need lived in long-stay wards in psychiatric hospitals. But since the 1950s successive governments have implemented a policy of closing these old psychiatric hospitals and providing as much care as possible outside hospital – in 'the community'. Many of the old hospitals or 'asylums' were built by the Victorians, and are sited outside towns. Usually, this gives them the advantages of spaciousness and large grounds. But their disadvantages tend to be inaccessibility, isolation from the rest of society and poor structural condition. In districts where an old asylum has been closed the general hospital in the main town usually contains psychiatric wards which are, in many ways, preferable. They are often in much better condition, more accessible, and more familiar. They are less likely than mental hospitals to attract prejudice and social stigma.

Community care is a sensible and humane strategy as long as everyone who needs inpatient care, or residential care, can have it. But there is a shortfall. The big problem with long-term community care at present is that demand exceeds supply. General hospital psychiatric units house far fewer psychiatric patients than the large Victorian asylums that they replaced. A typical asylum would have accommodated over 1000 patients at the turn of the century. Those old hospitals that now remain have 300–800 beds occupied, but the new units contain, on average, fewer than 100 beds. Researchers have shown that a number of homeless people have long-term mental illnesses and have somehow lost touch with psychiatric services. Many more have developed long-term problems, particularly related to alcohol, without ever getting in touch with psychiatric services.

One way of ensuring that everyone who needs long-term care is offered it is to assess all possible candidates thoroughly. After all, some may not need it for long, and some may not need it at all. The NHS and Community Care Act, passed in 1990, established a new breed of professionals called care managers to assess people whose long-term illnesses and disabilities make them unable to cope completely independently with life.[9] Care managers are given budgets by local councils to assess people's needs and arrange tailor-made packages of care, including services like home helps and day centres.

Since 1992 psychiatrists have had to ensure that people with severe mental illnesses have full programmes of care set up before discharge from hospital, to be overseen by named staff (key workers). A typical care programme for a young man with schizophrenia might include weekly visits at home from a community nurse, who gives him a monthly anti-psychotic injection, and regular check-ups with a psychiatrist at the outpatient clinic. For people who need intensive support from both health and social services, mental health key workers and social services care managers should work closely together. So for the man with schizophrenia, his care manager would arrange accommodation in a supervised communal home and social contact at a day centre, fitting in with the care programme as much as possible.

The community care arrangements may seem complicated, and for many sufferers, relatives, and friends guaranteed packages of care may sound like an expensive pipe dream. But there is plenty of evidence that community care can work and that it need not cost more than hospital care. For instance, the closures of two of the biggest mental hospitals in London have been carefully monitored and recorded by the Team for the Assessment of Psychiatric Services (the TAPS project), based at Friern Hospital in north London, and have progressed smoothly to community care. Critics of community care argue, however, that big projects like this are much better funded than most ordinary hospital closures. And they say that even one tragedy resulting from inadequate care, perhaps a suicide or even a homicide, should reverse the march to community care. And, according to one charity, the National Schizophrenia Fellowship, many of the 10–15 homicides a year carried out by people with severe mental illnesses result from inadequate community care.

1 ANXIETY AND RELATED PROBLEMS

Reacting to Stress

> I went to New York's great public library at Fifth Avenue and 42nd Street and discovered to my astonishment that this library had only 22 books listed under the title WORRY. I also noticed, to my amusement, that it had 189 books listed under WORMS. Almost nine times as many books about worms as about worry! Astounding, isn't it? Since worry is one of the biggest problems facing mankind, you would think, wouldn't you, that every high school and college in the land would give a course on 'How to stop worrying'?
>
> From *How to Stop Worrying and Start Living* by Dale Carnegie[1]

Since the 1940s, when Dale Carnegie wrote his bestseller, the number of books on worrying and how to stop it has mushroomed. But not all of them explain the nature of worry or stress and fewer still describe how to get professional help if worrying has got out of hand.

Of course, for most people, worrying does not usually get out of hand and feeling stressed is not necessarily a bad experience. Research has shown that people perform best in tests, for example doing calculations, when they are challenged and motivated by moderate stress. But above a certain threshold stress makes us feel uncomfortable, nervous, and unable to cope with the task presented. For example, actors usually need a degree of stage fright to stimulate a good performance. But if frozen with terror they might forget their lines, or even refuse to go onto the stage. This kind of sudden fear when anticipating a specific stressful event can be a nuisance and may occasionally be bad enough to warrant seeing a doctor.

More commonly, people seek help because they feel more worried about a certain source of stress than expected, given the circumstances. Sometimes the timing of symptoms is difficult to explain, occurring long after the event that initiated them or even completely out of the blue. For some the symptoms are too intense or persistent. And for many they make coping difficult, not only with stressful events, but also with other aspects of everyday life.

Doctors usually avoid the word stress, preferring terms that describe reactions to stress. This is mainly because the word is overused and non-specific, describing external problems as well as the internal experiences that those problems cause. 'Nerves', as in 'it's her nerves: they're terrible', does not mean much, either. The medical (but reassuringly untechnical) term for general symptoms of stress is anxiety. If it persists it is called an anxiety state, if it comes in sudden, overwhelming attacks it is called panic disorder.

Unbearable fear that can be dealt with only by avoiding the frightening stimulus is called a phobia. Phobic avoidance may be an acceptable response if the stimulus is encountered only rarely and the avoidance has little effect on life. Someone scared of heights, for example, is unlikely to seek medical help if the phobia only precludes rock climbing and holiday sightseeing from tall buildings. But the same phobia could be disastrous if it developed suddenly in a steeplejack. And some phobic sufferers become frightened of everyday events such as going to the shops and meeting people.

A much less common and more serious condition related to anxiety is obsessive-compulsive disorder. It starts with a specific form of worrying that is difficult to control: unwelcome ideas that intrude into ordinary thinking and usually compel the sufferer to take particular actions. Thus someone who is obsessionally worried about burglars might make a detailed check of the front door 20 times before going off to work, not quite convinced that it is safely locked. Such worries and actions may become so compelling that their interference with daily life becomes unbearable.

Many people who are stressed feel fed up and unable to enjoy life. This lowness of mood is sometimes so persistent and troubling that it amounts to depression. Because depression is such a big problem and takes so many forms, ranging from intense unhappiness to very serious mental illness, it has a chapter to itself in this book (see Chapter 2). Other common effects of feeling fed up and stressed include relationship problems, sexual problems, and certain physical complaints. All may need specialized help.

Although separating all these stress-related problems allows them to be described clearly, it implies that they are separate entities in real life. But they often occur together in varying proportions: for instance, someone may have a mixture of anxiety and depression with a few specific phobic symptoms. Doctors used to call all these conditions neuroses, but most psychiatrists now consider this general term too vague to be useful.

One recently recognized illness related to stress is also worth mentioning: post-traumatic stress disorder. Typically, it occurs after a single life-threatening event like an accident or mass disaster. The main symptoms are intrusive memories, dreams, and flashbacks that bring back the stressful event; avoidance of places, people and anything else that reminds the sufferer of the event; and a general feeling of anxiety and being on edge.

ANXIETY

Anxiety accounts for about one in ten of all new episodes of illness and about a third of all diagnosable psychiatric problems that a GP sees in a year. Many that do go to their doctors have vague physical problems, such as tiredness and indigestion, that may not be recognized as symptoms of anxiety.

According to the Department of Social Security, anxiety- and stress-related problems accounted for around half of the 92 million working days lost through mental illness in 1991.

The 1987 national Health and Lifestyle Survey, which looked at 9000 members of the British public, found that a third of the women and a quarter of the men had some symptoms of anxiety or depression or both. Other surveys suggest that about 3% of men and 4–5% of women suffer from persistent anxiety, like Ruth:

> Ruth's internal time clock seemed to have changed. She had been finding it difficult to get off to sleep at night, lying awake till the early hours with muddled thoughts churning around in her mind. In the mornings she found it difficult to wake up and was increasingly late for work, and once at the office she found concentration difficult. By the evenings she felt exhausted and could hardly face the housework and cooking.
>
> These symptoms had worsened so gradually that Ruth could not remember how or when they started. All she knew for sure was that it was at least six months since she had felt normal. There was no obvious explanation. Her elderly mother was a bit of a worry, and her teenage son was often difficult, but these problems seemed trivial in comparison with those of her friend who was coping admirably with a disabled husband. Ruth decided that she must just pull herself together. Perhaps she would feel better after the summer holiday.
>
> But Ruth continued to feel unwell and had such bad headaches in the afternoons that she was sent home early from work a couple of times and advised to see a doctor. But that seemed unnecessary, and she ignored the advice.
>
> One morning, standing in a crowded bus Ruth suddenly felt dizzy and sick. She felt terrified and convinced that she was going to collapse with a heart attack. There was a thumping in her chest, and a choking feeling in her throat. Unable to stand any longer, she pushed her way towards the door, stumbling past other passengers. One of them noticed how pale and ill she looked and shouted for the driver to stop urgently. Within half an

hour Ruth was sitting in the local hospital's casualty department, wired up to a heart monitor. It took the doctor another half an hour to convince her that there was nothing physically wrong, and that all her symptoms were caused by anxiety.

Signs and Symptoms of Anxiety

Anxiety can cause alarming physical symptoms like palpitations ('my heart races') and dizziness. Sufferers often go to their doctors because they fear they have heart disease or brain tumours. Many do not really recognize the psychological symptoms, assuming that they are just due to worry about being physically ill. The range of anxiety symptoms is summarized in Box 1.

BOX 1

Symptoms of anxiety

Psychological
- nervousness
- irritability
- worries (ruminations)
- insomnia and tiredness
- panic

Physical
- rapid pulse, pounding heart
- fast breathing
- aching and shaky limbs
- headache
- choking sensation
- sweaty skin, pale or flushed
- urges to urinate or open bowels

Psychological Symptoms

Most people with anxiety have strong feelings of nervousness and jumpiness. Some feel an uncomfortable anticipation, as if something unpleasant is about to happen. Irritability and short temper make them snappy. Inability to concentrate interferes with even simple tasks like reading a newspaper. These feelings usually worsen throughout the day.

Persistent worries, which doctors call ruminations, are common. Often they are not warranted. For example, an anxious person with a secure job and few current financial problems may dwell on the unlikely possibility of getting into serious debt. The experience is like that of Chicken Licken who thought that the sky might fall down in the well-known children's tale.

For many people who feel stressed, failure to sleep properly is the first sign that something is wrong. Transient insomnia at the time of exams or other well-defined events is a nuisance that only rarely needs treatment. But in anxiety states insomnia may persist and cause increasing tiredness. The typical pattern is difficulty in getting off to sleep (initial insomnia) followed by oversleeping in the morning.

The most alarming psychological symptom of anxiety is panic. The lay meaning of this word is obvious. Doctors describe panic as an explosive and self-perpetuating form of anxiety in which the fear of a particular situation is compounded by the fear of being afraid. Sufferers say they feel stuck in a whirl or spiral of rapidly increasing anxiety. For example, Ruth felt so anxious on the bus that she was sure that she was having a heart attack. In fact she was having a panic attack. The worse she felt physically, the worse she felt mentally, and so on. The severity of her symptoms spiralled upwards, way out of her control.

Physical Symptoms

Physical symptoms occur when the aroused mind in turn causes arousal of two main systems in the body, the autonomic nervous system and the skeletal muscles. The body has several systems of nerves, the most obvious being those that control our main muscles and five senses. But we are less aware of the more subtle control systems in the body, one of which is the autonomic (effectively automatic) nervous system.

The autonomic nervous system includes two distinct subsystems, the sympathetic and parasympathetic nerves, which control much of the body by the balanced effects of their opposing actions. Among the basic functions regulated by these nerves are the heartbeat, blood pressure, breathing rate, and digestion. When the mind is aroused by a threatening situation the autonomic nervous system quickly activates what scientists call the 'fight or flight' response. This response involves the release of chemicals into the blood, particularly the hormone adrenaline. In real danger, for example when faced with an assailant, the response may be life-saving. The main task is to provide the large muscles of the skeleton (particularly of the arms and legs) with the means to stand firm or run away. This causes a range of symptoms that can be very alarming if they occur in the absence of real external danger, during a panic attack.

Firstly, the pulse rate is increased, causing palpitations (thumping and fluttering feelings in the chest). This allows faster flow of blood through the muscles. Fast breathing increases the rate at which oxygen enters and the waste product carbon dioxide leaves the blood as it passes through the lungs. Thus the muscles can work more efficiently. But excessively fast breathing, called hyperventilation, can cause a chemical imbalance in the blood that in turn produces unpleasant symptoms. Although the body needs oxygen to function and finds carbon dioxide toxic in large quantities, some carbon dioxide is needed to help the brain gauge the normal breathing rate. When the breathing rate is increased by hyperventilation, too much carbon dioxide is exhaled and this in turn upsets the acidic balance in the blood. By a fairly simple chemical equation the blood concentration of calcium, a mineral, is reduced in an attempt to redress the balance. But sudden lack of calcium in the blood may cause numbness and tingling, particularly in the facial muscles round the mouth, and in extreme cases it can lead to jerky twitching of the wrists and hands ('I get nervous and out of breath, then pins and needles in my hands'). Needless to say, these symptoms are very alarming for the sufferer.

The blood supply to the muscles is increased further by diverting blood from the brain (causing light-headedness) and digestive tract (causing 'butterflies', nausea, and dry mouth). Changes in blood flow to the skin cause sweating and pallor, or sometimes flushing. External muscles tense up and feel odd with the increased blood supply. Poised for action, the arms and legs feel tense and may ache. The scalp and neck muscles may also hurt, causing headache ('The back of my neck gets achy and tense – then it spreads up to my head and down to the chest'). Tremors (shaking) and choking (caused by tension in the throat muscles) are particularly disturbing.

Internal muscles relax, and hence the bladder and bowels may want to open. All these symptoms go almost unnoticed when they occur in response to a real, immediate threat. But when they occur on their own they can feel like illness.

Causes of Anxiety
There is no single factor that always makes people anxious. Anxiety problems have several probable causes: some increase the risk of developing anxiety and some precipitate symptoms (see Box 2). Two underlying risk factors that have been studied in depth are inheritance and differences in brain function. Not surprisingly, life's stresses seem to be the main precipitating factor. Some physical illnesses, such as overactivity of the thyroid, include anxiety among their symptoms.

Whatever the cause of anxiety, experience tends to perpetuate it. When sufferers have to face situations in which they felt anxious previously, fear and anticipation increases the likelihood of another attack.

BOX 2

> **Probable causes of anxiety**
>
> *Risk factors*
> - Inheritance
> - Personality
> - Brain changes
>
> *Precipitating factors*
> - Stressful life events
> - Physical illness, e.g. thyroid overactivity, menopausal oestrogen deficiency, phaeochromocytoma
> - Withdrawal from addictive drugs, e.g. heroin, benzodiazepine tranquillizers

Inheritance

Anxiety states and panic attacks can affect anyone, not only those who are always shy and nervous. There is, however, some evidence of an inherited predisposition. Anxiety states affect about 15% of sufferers' close relatives compared with 3–5% in the general population. This difference in proneness to anxiety could be accounted for by upbringing.

But the genetic theory is supported by research in twins, performed in the 1960s and 70s. Among identical twins studied, sharing not only the same environment but also the same genes, over 40% of pairs suffered from anxiety states. Only 4% of non-identical twin pairs, who had the same environment but different genes, contained two sufferers. Curiously, this is considerably lower than the 15% reported for close relatives in general. The genetic theory of anxiety, therefore, is far from watertight.

Personality

Being nervous is an intrinsic part of some people's personalities ('My family always said I was a worrier'). Although being a born worrier does not automatically increase the risk of becoming unwell with anxiety, there is some evidence that anxious personalities are more likely than others to develop symptoms. Given that personality is partly inherited, this fits in with the genetic theory of anxiety.

Changes in the Brain

Research suggests that people suffering from severe anxiety have an excess of a chemical messenger (or neurotransmitter) called noradrenaline in one of the most primitive parts of the brain (the brainstem), which controls basic functions such as breathing. It is possible, but not confirmed, that vulnerability to these chemical changes is what is inherited.

Precipitating Factors

Stressful Life Events

One of the most basic stresses in life is change. Certain changes are particularly stressful – even apparently pleasant ones like getting married. Researchers in the United States looked at the medical notes of thousands of people and noticed that many of them mentioned getting married as a source of stress. The researchers decided to draw up a scale of stressful events, putting marriage in the middle with a score of 50 points.[2] Then they asked about 400 people of various ages and backgrounds to rate other common life events against marriage (Box 3).

BOX 3	*Life change scale (Holmes and Rahe 1967)*	
	Life event	*Score*
	Death of spouse	100
	Divorce	73
	Marital separation	65
	Jail term	63
	Death of close relative	63
	Injury or illness	53

Marriage	50
Being sacked	47
Marital reconciliation	45
Retirement	45
Change in health of close relative	44
Pregnancy	40
Sexual problems	39
Gaining a new family member	39
Change at work	39
Change in finances	38
Death of close friend	37
Change of career	36
Change in no. of arguments with spouse	35
Heavy mortgage	31
Defaulting on mortgage or loan	30
Changed responsibilities at work	29
Child leaving home	29
Trouble with in-laws	29
Outstanding personal achievement	28
Wife begins or stops work	26
Starting or leaving school	26
Change in living conditions	25
Change in habits (e.g. stopping smoking)	24
Trouble with boss	23
Changed working hours or conditions	20
Moving house	20
Moving schools	20
Change in recreation	19
Change in church activities	19
Change in social activities	18
Small mortgage	17
Change in sleeping habits	16
Change in no. of family get-togethers	15
Change in eating habits	15
Holiday	13
Christmas	12
Minor law-breaking	11

The researchers confirmed the common-sense assumption that more stress leads to more ill health. Of people who scored 200–300 points on the scale in one year, more than half had health problems in the next year, and nearly four-fifths of those who scored over 300 became ill. Some events tend to occur together; for example pregnancy usually entails changes in work, sex life, finances, sleeping habits, and size of family, accumulating nearly 200 points on the scale.

The scale gives a general idea of the kind of events that may cause stress and illness. Knowing that there might be a rough ride ahead could be helpful. Many of the changes on the list are self-inflicted, and anyone intending to make several of them at once might consider spreading out the load. Thus it might be unwise to change jobs just before getting married, if it is possible to wait a while.

Physical Illness

Some physical illnesses include anxiety among their symptoms or closely mimic it. Heart disease can cause a racing pulse and palpitations; lung problems such as asthma can cause breathlessness; and hormone imbalances can cause almost all anxiety symptoms. Hormones are chemical messengers that are made in glands and are carried round in the blood to tell other parts of the body what to do. The commonest hormone problem is lack of oestrogen during the menopause causing sweating, flushing, and sometimes anxiety. Thyroid gland overactivity and a rare non-cancerous growth that produces excess adrenaline in the adrenal gland (called a phaeochromocytoma) are other examples.

Withdrawal from Addictive Drugs

Addiction to alcohol (which some people may have without realizing it) can produce anxiety symptoms if the body misses a regular dose. And the full withdrawal syndromes that occur when addicts stop alcohol, heroin, and benzodiazepine tranquillizers (see p. 23) include anxiety.

Coping with Anxiety

Many people with anxiety cure it themselves. The first step is to look at all possible ways of reducing life's stressfulness. If the cause of anxiety symptoms is something transient, like exams, proper preparation can reduce the stress considerably. Doing enough work is obviously important, but it is not necessarily the only key to staying calm and passing. We all know people who sail through after what seems the minimum of revision, and others who study for months and still fail. Those who pass know how to learn and recall material systematically and how to keep cool.

These attributes may come partly from personality, but they can also be acquired through training. For exams there are many books that offer tips on technique. The main points in preparing for any transient but stressful event are shown in Box 4. Even if the anxiety-provoking event is more mundane, such as shopping, these tips can still help. Planning how long the trip will take, which shops to visit, what to buy and, most importantly, contingency plans in case these strategies go wrong, will all reduce the stress.

BOX 4

Preparing for brief stressful events, e.g. exams, public speaking

Find out as much as possible about what will happen (when, where, who with, how?)

Learn and rehearse the material in the same format that you will have to perform it in on the day, e.g. learn for written papers by preparing essay plans on the core subjects, practise a speech in front of a mirror

Predict what could go wrong, e.g. dry mouth while speaking (ask for water), pen running out during exam (take spares)

Visit the venue in advance, practise the journey there

Ask a friend to accompany you there on the day

If there is an obvious cause for the anxiety but it is long-lasting, like one of the persistent life changes in the Holmes and Rahe scale (see pp. 10–11), more general strategies are needed to avoid excessive stress (see Box 5). Insomnia is particularly hard to deal with, but the self-help methods listed in Box 6 are often effective.

BOX 5

How to reduce long-term stress

- Try to enjoy life more and allow time for recreation

- Share your problems and feelings with others

- Do not avoid stressful situations unless they are unimportant – they will be harder to face later and you will become phobic (see pp. 26–33)

- Get to know your stress threshold beyond which you will perform badly

- Do not make too many life changes at once – expect to feel stressed if you cannot avoid major change

- Learn to relax – try yoga or a relaxation tape

- Be kind to your body – eat healthily, exercise

- Do not drink too much alcohol (see Chapter 5)

- Do not drink more than five cups of coffee or cola a day – both contain stimulant drugs that can cause anxiety

- Get enough sleep

BOX 6

How to beat insomnia

During the day

- avoid naps, even if you feel exhausted
- exercise, e.g. walk instead of driving
- avoid stimulants (coffee, tea, cola) after 6 p.m.

Before bed

- take a warm bath
- have a warm milky drink (without caffeine)

In bed

- read, listen to music
- leave a low light on
- relax – try autohypnosis
  (a) close your eyes and imagine you can see the huge word SLEEP, perhaps carved from rock. Trace out in your mind every contour of the big 3-D letters in detail;
  (b) if you wake in the night and cannot get back to sleep within 30 minutes get up and do something – reading, ironing, watching TV. Don't lie there worrying. Go back to bed when tired again.

Coping with Panic Attacks

The most important fact for sufferers to remember if panic strikes is that the symptoms are nothing more than an exaggeration of the normal reaction to sudden stress, and are not harmful. This is half the battle because it stops the panic spiral. Understanding what is happening in the body reduces worry about what might happen.

Distraction, thinking of something else that is completely unrelated to the situation, will reduce anxiety. Focusing on other people's conversations, shop window displays, the contents of a handbag or wallet, or a bus timetable – these are all simple sources of distraction. If the symptoms are too strong to be swamped by these external distractions they may succumb to mental exercises like counting up to 100 and back or reciting a favourite poem.

Hyperventilation (see p. 7) is one of the most frightening symptoms of panic. The best way to beat it is to use deep breathing exercises as soon as the panic starts: breathing through the nose in a rhythm, counting to four when breathing in and to eight on breathing out. In an emergency, if concentrating on deep breathing is impossible, the chemical imbalance in the blood can be controlled by altering the gases breathed in. This is done very simply by breathing in and out of a paper (NOT plastic) bag, recycling the same air and thereby increasing the amount of carbon dioxide in the blood. The bag should be bunched up and held over the mouth and nose so that no air leaks out. As long as the bag is kept there for several minutes, the chemistry of the blood will make the breathing centre in the brain slow down to a normal rate. This may look a bit daft, but it really works. And it is quite safe – paper lets some gases in and out and will not allow suffocation, unlike plastic.

Understanding these symptoms takes away the fear of being afraid. There is one other important thing to do: staying in the same place until the anxiety goes. Running away will just make facing the same situation much harder in future. Knowing that the panic can be controlled, on the other hand, will make the next time a lot easier to cope with.

Getting Specialized Help

Relaxation Training
Relaxation does not come naturally to everyone. But it can be learnt in classes or from audio tapes and videos, most of which are based on a 60-year-old technique called Jacobsen's progressive muscular relaxation. In essence, students of this technique must lie down quietly in a warm comfortable place

slowly tense and relax each group of muscles in the body in turn (see Box 7).

BOX 7

Relaxation training

Relaxation exercises are directed by the slow, calm voice of a teacher, starting like this:

Lie on your back with arms by your side, palms upwards, and eyes closed.

Concentrate on what I am saying.

Aim to become increasingly aware of the sensations in your body. You cannot feel relaxed if your mind is intent on making decisions or solving problems.

Please concentrate on your breathing. Use as much of your lungs as you can, in a rhythmic pattern of breathing. As you breathe in, try to imagine that every part of your body is energized, and as you breathe out imagine that your tension flows away.

Point your right foot away from your body – hold it there as long as possible – then relax.

Curl the toes up towards your body – hold it – and relax.

Point your left foot away from your body . . .

The exercises work slowly up to the face and usually end like this:

Screw up your face into a tight ball – hold it – relax.

Stretch your face – hold it – relax.

Think about your breathing. It should be deep and rhythmic.

As you lie there I will recap. If part of your body does not feel relaxed when I mention it, concentrate on relaxing it now.

Feet and calves should feel relaxed. Pause.
Thighs and hips should feel relaxed. Pause.
Bottom and stomach should feel relaxed. Pause.
Back and chest should feel relaxed. Pause.
Shoulders and neck should feel relaxed. Pause.
Arms and hands should feel relaxed. Pause.
Head and face should feel relaxed. Pause.

I will now play some music. Imagine you are lying on a soft white cloud, feeling warm, comfortable, and relaxed.

The session ends with a piece of gentle music. While it is playing, participants gradually sit, then stand up. The session is over.

The most useful part of relaxation training is learning how muscular tension feels. It is possible to sit all day at a desk with tense, hunched shoulders or to drive for miles while gripping the steering wheel tightly and not even be aware of the muscular work involved. Because relaxation training shows what muscles feel like when they are tense, its students find it easier to relax at any time – not only when listening to a tape at home. Thus, someone standing in a bus queue can deliberately loosen tense muscles just by realizing that they are tense; yet the nearest person in the queue will not even notice.

Relaxation tapes can be bought for a few pounds in most bookshops, and local classes are commonly held in church halls and community centres. The local library may have a list. An organization that can recommend teachers is Relaxation for Living (see Appendix 2).

Counselling and Psychotherapy
Some anxious people with specific worries may prefer to pay a private counsellor than to discuss their underlying problems with friends and relatives. Even a few half hour counselling sessions, aimed at solving problems (for example, learning to adjust to one of the life changes described earlier) may do the trick. If the cause of the anxiety seems to be deep-rooted, and the anxious person feels able to talk in depth about feelings and past experiences, more specialized psychotherapy may be appropriate.

The National Association for Mental Health (MIND) and the British Association for Counselling (see Appendix 2 for addresses) can recommend counsellors. GPs and mental health centres can suggest where to get counselling, and some will even provide it, along with a range of more specialized treatments. Elements and sources of psychotherapy are discussed in detail in the Introduction.

Treatments for Anxiety and Panic
The first thing doctors should do when a patient complains of anxiety is to confirm the diagnosis. If physical anxiety symptoms are prominent the GP may perform some health checks to make sure that there is no other cause such as thyroid disease. A full examination and some simple tests may be necessary.

Knowing that anxiety is the only problem may prove so reassuring that no other help will be necessary. But some people do need more, and they can get both psychological and physical treatments (drugs) through their GPs (see Box 8).

BOX 8

Treatments for anxiety

Psychological
- Counselling and psychotherapy
- Anxiety management training
- Social skills training

Physical (drugs)
- Beta-blockers
- Antidepressants
- Tranquillizers

Psychological Treatments for Anxiety
Psychological treatments for anxiety are available in some general practice health centres. Referral to a specialist is the alternative, and it may be necessary anyway if the problems are too severe for health centre staff to manage. Specialists might be psychologists, psychiatrists, psychiatric nurses, occupational therapists, or social workers. They may work in mental health centres, hospital clinics, GPs' surgeries, or even in patients' homes. Treatment options include counselling and psychotherapy (as above), behaviour therapy, and social skills training.

Behaviour therapy is just what it sounds like: a way to alter unwanted or unpleasant behaviour. A special kind of behaviour therapy called anxiety management training is widely available through local health and social services. Typically a course of this training will run for eight weeks. People who enrol, usually with six to eight others in a group, must attend each session to get the greatest benefit because each session is different. An outline of how an anxiety management course changes behaviour is shown in Box 9. One of the greatest benefits of group training is meeting other people with similar problems, so that sufferers realize that they are not alone.

BOX 9

Anxiety management training sessions

1 Learn about the symptoms of anxiety, both mental and physical
2 Identify situations causing anxiety and prepare for them
3 Learn special ways to cope with symptoms – for example relaxation training, distraction techniques, and positive thinking
4 Discuss how anxiety affects life and set goals to stop its effects
5 Learn to accept anxiety as a natural response that everyone experiences at times
6 Improve self-esteem by discussing achievements so far
7 Discuss how to apply these techniques in future, without support of group

Each session starts with recapping and reporting on progress with practical home-work set at the end of the previous meeting.

Some people become particularly anxious when having to meet and socialize with others. This may come from inherent shyness or may be part of an anxiety state. But such problems can be overcome by social skills training, which is becoming increasingly available (see Box 10 for outline). After all, skills for communication and socializing are not completely inbred, they are normally learnt by trial and error. General practice health centres, mental health centres, and social services departments should have details of local groups.

BOX 10 | **Social Skills Training**

This group therapy shows people:

- How communication depends on body language as well as words
- How social interactions work. Therapists act out examples
- How to act out the same situations on video to get feedback
- How to improve social skills, particularly body language
- How to practise the new skills in real life

Drug Treatment for Anxiety

Three main groups of drugs can help to reduce anxiety. But all drugs have some unwanted effects, and certain tranquillizers used to treat anxiety have caused considerable problems, including addiction. Now that the risks of such drugs are clear and psychological treatments have become more widely available, doctors should not routinely prescribe medicines as the first line of treatment. None the less, drugs can still help in emergencies, perhaps when bereavement causes acute anxiety or when a severely anxious person is waiting for psychological treatment. Some doctors prescribe them in advance to cover specific stressful events like exams or public speaking engagements.

Perhaps the best drugs for anxiety are the beta-blockers. Their full name is the beta adrenoceptor blocking drugs because they bind to special sites on the nerves of the sympathetic nervous system (see p. 7). The sites, called beta adrenoceptors, receive chemical messages that stimulate the nerves into action – increasing blood pressure, making the pulse and heartbeat race, and causing tremors. Beta-blockers stop these chemical messages and thereby reduce the nerves' actions. They are most commonly used to treat high blood pressure and heart problems. But they also reduce the physical symptoms of anxiety.

Beta-blockers do not tranquillize or sedate. They reduce fear and worry indirectly by interrupting the physical spiral of panic. The anxious person then has to deal only with the primary worries, and not the extra ones induced by frightening physical symptoms. Beta-blockers can also reduce persistent headache, particularly migraine.

Like all drugs, however, beta-blockers have some disadvantages. Firstly, they should not be given to people with asthma, chronic bronchitis, certain kinds of heart disease, or circulatory problems in the legs, and they may upset the control of blood glucose in diabetic people. Secondly, side effects in otherwise healthy people occasionally include wheezing, bowel upsets, and impotence (failure of erection). Lastly, although beta-blockers are not addictive, they must be tailed off slowly at the end of treatment because they can cause a rebound increase in blood pressure if stopped suddenly.

Antidepressant drugs may be prescribed for anxiety. There are two reasons for this. Firstly, many people with anxiety are also depressed: feelings of fearfulness may not go away until the mood lifts. Secondly, some drugs in this family are sedating in small doses. None of them is addictive. Chapter 2, on depression, discusses antidepressants in detail.

Tranquillizers, despite their great efficacy, have a limited role in treating anxiety because they have proved over the years to be very addictive. About 30 years ago, a new family of tranquillizing drugs promised to revolutionize the treatment of anxiety. They were called benzodiazepines and the best known examples were diazepam (trade name Valium), nitrazepam (Mogadon), lorazepam (Ativan), and chlordiazepoxide (Librium). In testing and early use these drugs seemed to overcome all the problems that were becoming obvious with their highly addictive predecessors, the barbiturates.

Benzodiazepines are extremely effective tranquillizers. Some sedate and stop insomnia, others induce less sleepiness but simply produce an unworried calm. Over the past ten years, however, severe addictions to benzodiazepines have developed and now they are recommended for only short-term use (see Box 11). The guidelines shown here come from a detailed report on benzodiazepine use in general practice drawn up by and available from the Mental Health Foundation (see directory in Appendix 2 for address). The foundation is a charity that raises awareness of and funding for mental health and provides grants for research.

BOX 11

> **Mental Health Foundation's guidelines on short-term treatment with benzodiazepine tranquillizers**
>
> - Benzodiazepines should be reserved for anxiety which is severe and disabling, or for severe insomnia
> - They should be given for no more than four weeks for anxiety
> - They should be given for no more than one week for insomnia

A MORI poll commissioned in 1984 by the BBC television consumer programme *That's Life* found that up to a quarter of a million people in Britain were addicted to tranquillizers prescribed by doctors. Almost 10 million people, 23% of the population, had taken tranquillizers at some time and of them a quarter had taken the drugs continuously for more than a year. At the same time *That's Life* and MIND (the National Association for Mental Health) jointly surveyed over 2000 viewers who were taking tranquillizers. In the second survey, two-thirds had taken the drugs continuously for at least five years and more than three-quarters of the total sample said they had been addicted, unable to stop the drugs without a fight.[3] Further information and advice on tranquillizers can be obtained from MIND, whose address is listed in Appendix 2.

Addiction to benzodiazepine drugs is treatable. This usually entails careful reduction of the drug over several weeks or even months, depending on the period of previous usage.

Sometimes a less addictive benzodiazepine is used as a substitute that can then be reduced gradually. While the tranquillizers are slowly withdrawn, psychological treatment may be needed for the anxiety that will probably emerge again. Practical advice on benzodiazepine addiction can be found in Shirley Trickett's book *Coming Off Tranquillizers and Sleeping Tablets*.[4]

One other problem has arisen with tranquillizers. A benzodiazepine sleeping pill called triazolam (trade name Halcion) was banned in Britain in 1991 after reports that it had caused violent behaviour among people using it in the USA. In 1993 the drug's manufacturers took the British government to court to contest the ban, citing evidence from two scientific panels who said that Halcion was no different from other benzodiazepines that were still available.

Finally, there are a few other drugs that may be prescribed for anxiety, including a new one called buspirone (trade name Buspar). It seems to be effective but it has not been available long enough to be deemed completely non-addictive. Its manufacturers say it should not be given during pregnancy or breastfeeding because its effects on the baby are not yet known. They also say that people taking Buspar should avoid alcohol.

The main point about drugs for anxiety is that they are not usually necessary. People offered anti-anxiety drugs by their doctors should think twice and ask for more information before agreeing to such treatment.

Outcome of Treatment for Anxiety

Two-thirds of the people who see doctors about severe anxiety states improve substantially or recover. For those whose symptoms persist (often those who see the problem as entirely physical and do not recognize the need to reduce levels of psychological stress), treatment usually improves the ability to cope with social situations.

If anxiety does persist, there is reassuring evidence that it does not predispose sufferers to serious mental illness. Rates of schizophrenia and manic depressive illness are just as low among anxious patients followed up as in the general population. But there is a greater risk of other common psychiatric problems like phobias and mild depression, and indeed, such problems often appear at the same time. Mild mixed problems usually clear up within six months and only about one in twenty-five sufferers stays ill for as long as three years.

PHOBIAS, OBSESSIONS, AND COMPULSIONS

Phobias are fears of particular situations that do not normally bother most people. Even though the feeling is unreasonable because there is no real danger, the fear causes such intense anxiety that the only way of coping is to leave the situation or avoid it altogether. The symptoms of anxiety are just as described earlier in this chapter and may be so bad that they amount to panic.

The commonest phobias are of people, either in mass gatherings (agoraphobia) or in everyday social situations (social phobia). Agoraphobia is sometimes described as a fear of open spaces, but this gives the misleading impression that it could occur in the middle of an empty field. The Greek word for market place is agora, and a crowded square full of noisy, bustling people is just the kind of situation that would really provoke anxiety in an agoraphobic person. The modern-day equivalent is a supermarket ('I was in the checkout queue when I felt hot and sweaty, my knees felt like they would give way and I had to go and sit down or else I thought I would faint'). Social phobia is often prompted by having to meet people in ordinary everyday situations, not only in obviously demanding circumstances such as formal social occasions. Other common provokers of phobias are more specific, such as darkness, thunderstorms, enclosed spaces, heights, snakes, and spiders. Many people have mild versions of these phobias but few need to seek medical help.

Closely related to phobias are obsessions. These are spontaneous intrusive thoughts that cause anxiety. They can arise at any time and are not triggered by particular situations. The thoughts may comprise single, repetitive words or phrases, internal arguments, doubts like 'did I shut the front door when I came to work today?' or vividly imagined scenes, for example of something distressing like a road accident. Because the resulting feelings are uncomfortable, the thinker tries to dispel the obsessional thoughts but fails. Many of the thoughts prompt urges, or compulsions, to perform certain acts. Thus the problem is called obsessive-compulsive disorder.

Someone with this disorder, for example a clerical worker, might have an unwarranted fear that a piece of paperwork has not been done properly. This fear will compel the clerk to keep checking the relevant file, even if the previous five checks in the past hour have shown that the work has been done. Such a compulsive act may become so entrenched that it takes on the quality of a senseless ritual that is far removed from any logical explanation ('I knew it was stupid but I just couldn't stop checking').

Rituals are often seen in normal childhood but they are usually transient and harmless. Avoiding cracks in the pavement to stop bears eating you up is a common example, reinforced by myth and fiction. In adulthood compulsive rituals are nearly always unwelcome. Some are harmful. For example, a sufferer from obsessive-compulsive disorder may get an urge to wash their hands repeatedly until they are cracked and sore because of a persistent but illogical conviction that they have become contaminated. Other, less disruptive, examples include meaningless checking to see whether things are in the right place: handles on furniture drawers must be perfectly in line with each other, and clothes must be hung in a certain order in the wardrobe.

Phobias and obsessive-compulsive disorder are surprisingly common. They probably occur to a disabling degree in about one in twenty of the population, although only a few sufferers seek help. These problems are commoner in women than men, and usually start to become a nuisance in young adulthood.

Causes of Phobias, Obsessions, and Compulsions

All these problems are thought to arise from an abnormal and powerful kind of learning. In theory, people who have felt very anxious in certain situations in the past suffer greater and greater anxiety each time they have to face similar situations and fail to deal with them satisfactorily. From each experience like this they learn, subconsciously, to react anxiously (and phobically or obsessively) at certain times.

Simple phobias may be remnants from childhood. Fear of dogs, for example, may spring from a bad experience such as being bitten. Fear can be picked up from others too; often from parents.

Agoraphobia and social phobia usually develop from general anxiety and have the same underlying causes as anxiety. The phobic symptoms, however, come from avoiding the source of anxiety. For instance a panic attack in a shop may be so terrifying that avoidance of that shop and others like it seems the only way to stop it happening again. When the sufferer has to go shopping again the resulting anxiety is doubled by anticipation, and the urge to avoid the experience in future is amplified still further.

Obsessional anxiety may have a separate constitutional origin in addition to a history of anxiety-associated learning. As is mentioned below, certain antidepressant drugs are thought to be specifically active in treating severe obsessional symptoms. These drugs have effects on one particular brain chemical system, the 5HT, or serotonin system. These treatment results have led to the belief that obsessional disorder, unlike most other anxiety-related problems, is specifically a disorder of the serotonin system.

Coping with Phobias, Obsessions and Compulsions

Firstly, all the ways of coping with anxiety that were described earlier should help. After all, anxiety is a large part of the problem. Most importantly, the cause of the phobic or obsessive anxiety must be faced. This is much easier than it sounds if it is done very gradually in manageable steps. Carol, who had a phobia, managed to face her fear without professional help:

> Carol was frightened of spiders but she did not see this as a real problem. If she found one in the bath, she would ask someone else to move it and then forget about it. But one morning, while driving to work on the other side of London, Carol saw a large spider on the floor of her car in front of the passenger seat. She tried to keep calm, telling herself that the tiny creature was harmless. But, despite having the radio at full blast, she could not keep her mind off the spider and began to feel increasingly anxious. There was no point in stopping and trying to move the spider. She could not bring herself to touch it. The only option was to get someone else to move it.
>
> Carol's sense of embarrassment prevented her from flagging down a stranger, so she decided to get to work and find a friend to help her. Barely able to concentrate, she drove much too quickly, and only just avoided an accident. By the time she reached work she was panicking. Her heart was racing and she was breathless, dizzy, and terrified. At last she found a friend who moved the offending spider and took her off to the coffee room to calm down. As she recovered from her panic, Carol resolved never to repeat the experience.
>
> That lunchtime Carol started her treatment. She went out and bought a book on spiders, one with large photographs that made her shudder. Little by little over the next few days, she progressed from reading the text to looking long and hard at the illustrations, until she felt quite comfortable with the book. The next stage was to confront a real spider.
>
> Several trips to London Zoo were necessary before Carol could bear to look at the captive spiders. But eventually she was able to study even the largest tropical species through the glass. Finally, a friend caught and placed in a jar a large household spider. Carol gave it

a pet name and gradually learned to feed it and pick up its jar quite easily. After a few days she let it go in the garden. The next time she found a spider in the bath she put a glass over it, slid a piece of paper under the glass and put the spider outside. She felt fine.

Carol's problem may sound small, but her story is true and her problem might have become quite disabling if she had not confronted it. The general principle of facing fear is the key to treating all phobias. Obsessions and compulsions can also be confronted. But obsessional ideas and the anxiety that accompanies them are usually so strong that self-help in this way is difficult. An easier way to cope with such ideas is to block them out. A well-rehearsed poem, song, or just a list of numbers can be recited under the breath as a distraction whenever the unwanted ideas start to intrude. Some sufferers find physical distractions more effective, for instance by wearing a rubber band round the wrist and flicking it against the skin. The principle is the same as pinching yourself to stay awake and to avoid nodding off at an awkward moment.

Further information on phobias and obsessions is available from the sources shown in Box 12.

BOX 12	**Phobias and Obsessions**
	Help and further information are available from:
	*Organizations**
	The Phobics Society
	Phobic Action
	The Maudsley Hospital

* See Appendix 2 for addresses

Books

Living with Fear by Isaac Marks (McGraw Hill, 1978)

Who's Afraid of Agoraphobia? by Alice Neville (Century Hutchinson Arrow, 1986)

Agoraphobia by Claire Weekes (Angus and Robertson, 1984)

Treatments for Phobias, Obsessions and Compulsions

The first step a doctor should make is to confirm the diagnosis. The specific symptoms of phobic and obsessive-compulsive disorder are easy to recognize, however, so checking for hidden physical illness may not be necessary. Referral for specialized help is the next step.

Behaviour therapy is the mainstay of treatment for phobias and obsessive-compulsive problems. As Carol worked out for herself, the key to treating phobias and obsessions is to face the fear gradually and learn to respond to it more calmly and rationally. In other words, controlled exposure to the fear during therapy leads to a change in behaviour. Logically enough, this kind of behaviour therapy is called exposure therapy. Its essence is helping the sufferer to write down a programme of tasks to be worked through one by one (see Box 13). For example, a therapist would help an agoraphobic person to work out a programme of gradual steps that lead to the local shopping centre, starting with a walk to the garden gate.

BOX 13 **Exposure Therapy for Phobias**

A therapist and an agoraphobic person will agree on a written programme like this:

1. Aim: to enable the person to go out alone

2. Method: to devise a graded programme of trips from home, for example:

- to garden gate (5m from front door)
- to letter box (20m from home)
- to post office (50m)
- to bus stop (100m), etc

3. Rules: each trip must be taken in turn

- the therapist will accompany the agoraphobic person

- the patient will persevere with each trip until anxiety dies down

- each trip must be completed before starting the next

- if a trip cannot be completed because of anxiety it will be broken down into smaller steps

- feelings aroused will be discussed so that the therapist can advise and encourage the agoraphobic person

---

In obsessive-compulsive disorder exposure therapy is usually used to desensitize the sufferer gradually, but occasionally a more sudden method called flooding is used. A compulsive hand washer obsessed by unwarranted fears of contamination can overcome fear by getting dirty hands and seeing that no great harm follows. This should be done only with a therapist who can help to deal with the severe anxiety that will probably ensue.

People with compulsive rituals often need one additional technique: response prevention. The therapist will help the patient to overcome the urge to perform the ritual. Initially this will involve delaying the ritual for a few minutes, eventually treatment will stop it completely. This may mean physical intervention at first, such as holding the hands of a compulsive washer so that he or she cannot wash them.

Two antidepressant drugs called clomipramine (Anafranil)

and fluoxetine (Prozac) may help in both phobic and obsessive-compulsive disorders, even when the commonly accompanying depression is not present. These drugs may have a direct effect on thinking and behaviour that is not part of their antidepressant action. They are normally needed for several months. They are not addictive.

Outcome of Exposure Therapy

About 85% of people who start exposure therapy complete it and two-thirds obtain considerable relief from it, even those with long-term illness. At London's Maudsley Hospital a special behaviour therapy unit for inpatients treats people referred from all over Britain. People with obsessive-compulsive disorder who were contacted six months after treatment at the unit in 1988 and 1989 said that they were spending, on average, four-fifths less time each day on compulsive rituals.[5] Most said that they now had much more time for work, leisure, and social life. Their relatives felt much less burden, too.

PROBLEMS WITH RELATIONSHIPS, SEX AND GENERAL HEALTH

The boundaries often get blurred between stress-related illnesses like anxiety and personal problems involving relationships, sex, and general health. Sometimes anxiety arises from these problems, sometimes it causes them.

Relationship Problems

Relationship problems are all too common and are an underlying cause of many psychiatric symptoms. Medical and psychiatric help is mostly too specialized for problems directly involving a relationship. Help is available though, in the form of counselling.

The most widespread source of relationship counselling is the organization Relate, which has branches all over Britain. Relate's trained volunteers will consider helping anyone with a relationship problem; whether married or single, heterosexual or homosexual, in couples or alone. This broad approach, dealing with much more than the problems of marriage, is one reason why the organization changed its name from the Marriage Guidance Council. After an initial assessment interview there may be a waiting list of a couple of months to see a counsellor. Counselling takes place during up to 10 weekly hour-long sessions. Relate does not charge fees but welcomes and depends on donations.

Now that many gay men and women who openly declare their sexual orientation are plainly psychologically healthy, the concept of homosexuality as an illness is outdated. Most psychiatrists now view sexual orientation as a choice, and recognize that many people try both homosexual and heterosexual experiences at different times of their lives. The theory was complicated in 1993 by the discovery that a tendency for men to be homosexual seems to be inherited via part of the X chromosome. (The normal genetic blueprint for humans includes 43 pairs of chromosomes in each cell. One of these pairs determines gender: women have a pair of X chromosomes, men have an X from their mothers and a Y from their fathers.)

Regardless of genetic predisposition, sexual orientation still seems to be partly a matter of choice. Surveys show that about 33% of American men and about 6% of women have had homosexual experiences leading to orgasm at some time in their lives, mainly during adolescence.[6] Even though homosexuality is common, prejudice in society can make it a difficult choice. And although gay people with relationship problems can contact Relate and other general counselling organizations, some prefer to know that they are talking to someone with the same sexual orientation. Most large towns in Britain have phone helplines for gay people, advertised in local phone directories. Gay Switchboard's national office, whose address and phone number is given in the directory (Appendix 2), can also help.

Practical Sexual Problems
Common sexual problems include premature ejaculation for men and difficulty in reaching orgasm for women (see Box 14). Most of these physical problems have psychological causes such as anxiety, so they are called psychosexual problems.

BOX 14

> **Psychosexual problems[7]**
>
> Affecting sexual desire
> - reduced libido (lack of interest in sex)
>
> Impairing arousal
> - erectile impotence (complete or partial inability to get and maintain erection)
> - lack of vaginal lubrication
>
> Impairing orgasm
> - premature ejaculation (sooner than both partners wish)
> - retrograde ejaculation (sperm goes into bladder, usually after prostate surgery)
> - elusive or absent female orgasm
>
> Causing pain
> - vaginismus (powerful constriction of muscles in vaginal wall)
> - pain in vagina or pelvis during sex
> - pain on ejaculation

There is little information on how often psychosexual problems occur. One specialist clinic checked its records and worked out that about 0.6% of the local adult population attended for help each year. But this figure undoubtedly represents only the tip of the iceberg. Typical clients attending specialist psychosexual clinics are heterosexual couples in which both partners have a problem. In about a third of couples the problems are loss of libido for the woman and premature ejaculation for the man. Studies suggest that 6% of men suffer premature ejaculation at some time, increasing with age. Kinsey's famous American survey in the late 1940s showed persistent impotence among 1.3% of men under 35, 6.7% under 50 and 18.4% under 60.[8]

Expectations about sex and levels of desire vary and usually (but not always) lessen with age. There is no such thing as a normal sexual frequency, despite jokes and boasts among friends about the number of times a week that intercourse takes place. The same applies for sexual styles and preferences. What really matters is that both partners are comfortable and happy with the sexual part of their relationship; even if they choose to be celibate. Persistent unhappiness about sex can be very destructive to relationships and is worth trying to sort out.

As with so many problems in life, half the battle against sexual difficulties can be won simply by talking. Even if talking fails to find a cause for the problem it can make couples feel closer again. But many couples find frank discussion difficult. Apart from emotional barriers such as embarrassment and guilt, practical problems get in the way. Married people with children may be able to spare only a few minutes each week in meaningful discussion.

Whatever the sexual problem, it will be lessened by trying to recapture some of the pleasure of the early days of the relationship. When couples first get together they tend to spend time kissing and talking intimately as part of the cementing of the relationship. And they may not restrict their sex lives to bed or to the night. If you think about it, it's amazing that any tired couple feels sexy on getting into bed at the end of a long hard day. If the problem has not yet turned both partners right off the idea of sex, varying the time and place for sex can rekindle desire. Relaxation helps too; using music, massage, or a relaxation tape. Alcohol, however, is not a reliable relaxant. Tipsiness can make people feel laid back and amorous, but being drunk notoriously hampers short-term performance (particularly erection) and regular heavy drinking can cause long-term harm. Heavy smoking, too, can reduce the male sexual response.

There are many books and videos explaining sex and sexual problems in detail, and others that also cover wider aspects of women's and men's problems. *Everywoman: A Gynaecological Guide for Life* and *Everyman*, both by Derek Llewellyn-Jones, a former consultant obstetrician and gynaecologist, are particularly informative.[9]

If self-help is not enough, direct professional advice and treatment for psychosexual problems can be arranged by the Family Planning Information Service (see Appendix 2 for address) or by GPs. Before arranging counselling or behaviour therapy, however, a doctor should check that the sexual problem is not caused by an undiagnosed physical problem. When doctors ask about early morning erections, masturbation, or sex with other partners they are not prying, but are trying to see how much of the sexual function is affected. Physical examination may include the nervous system and circulation as well as the genitals, and blood pressure should be checked. Men having difficulty with erection may have to provide urine and blood specimens to test for diabetes because this illness can affect the nerve supply to the penis. Other physical illnesses, and certain drugs, that can affect sexual function are summarized in Boxes 15 and 16.

BOX 15	*Physical illnesses that can reduce sexual function*	
	Hormonal	diabetes, thyroid disease, Addison's disease (a disorder of the adrenal glands)
	Gynaecological	vaginal, pelvic, and uterine infections; vaginal dryness; endometriosis (growth of uterine cells outside uterus with pain and period problems)

Heart disease	angina (chest pain on exertion), previous heart attack, long-term high blood pressure
Lung disease	asthma, chronic bronchitis
Skeletal	arthritis, back pain
Kidney disease	kidney failure
Neurological	paraplegia, multiple sclerosis

BOX 16

Drugs that can reduce sexual function
Alcohol

Nicotine

Antihypertensives and diuretics (for high blood pressure)

Antidepressants

Tranquillizers

Antipsychotic drugs

Some pain killers (mainly for arthritis)

Steroid hormones (for contraception, hormone replacement, some cancers)

Specialist psychosexual treatment involves two main approaches, counselling and behaviour therapy. Counselling has three main aims: to dispel any myths and unhelpful attitudes about sex, to increase communication between partners, and to set goals for treatment. If the main reason for sexual difficulties is a long-term psychological or mental health problem the psychosexual therapist may advise psychotherapy or treatment elsewhere.

The main treatment approach used in psychosexual clinics is a form of behaviour therapy based on the work of two researchers, Masters and Johnson, in the 1970s. The idea is that most psychosexual problems develop from loss of confidence in or anxiety about performance. Most sex therapy, therefore, involves a series of graded tasks or exercises to do at home. This is called sensate focus therapy. The therapist (or therapists: often two together) will start by banning intercourse for the time being. This takes the heat off and dispels the feeling that any caress or kiss must lead straight to sex. The tasks are sessions of kissing and caressing (initially anywhere but the genitals) in which partners take it in turns to please each other. The tasks slowly build up to the desired end point, usually full intercourse. But intercourse happens only when the therapist, who sees the couple regularly, is happy that they are ready.

Kingsley Amis gives a good, if somewhat flippant, description of sensate focusing therapy in his book *Jake's Thing*:

> 'What does it mean?' asked Brenda.
>
> 'Well, sensate ought to mean endowed with sense or senses, as dentate if it occurs means endowed with teeth, but I don't see how any sort of focusing can be endowed with any sort of sense. I think they wanted an adjective from sense and noticed or someone told them sensuous and sensual were used up and they noticed or someone told them a lot of words ended in -ate. Makes it sound scientific too. Like nitrate. And focusing, well. Homing in on? No? Concentrating? Something like that.'
>
> 'I see. But what does it mean?'
>
> 'Christ, love, I don't know. Getting you, getting one interested in the other person physically, something like that I should think . . .'[10]

Certain psychosexual problems respond well to specific sex therapies as well as or instead of sensate focusing. For example, women whose partners do not bring them to orgasm, or do not have them at all, can learn to climax by using a vibrator. And premature ejaculation can be prevented by the alarming-sounding but harmless technique of squeezing the penis tightly for a few seconds when ejaculation seems imminent. This takes away the desire to ejaculate until later, after much longer stimulation.

Psychosexual therapy may sound unbearably embarrassing, but it is well worth trying. Therapists are usually unembarrassable, with a warm sense of humour, and sessions at clinic can be quite entertaining once initial inhibitions are overcome. The homework can be fun, too. Couples often come back to the clinic with cheerful thanks, saying that their whole relationship has improved. At least two-thirds of psychosexual problems can be cured by counselling and behaviour therapy. Success usually depends on the couple's motivation and on the quality of their general relationship.

Stress-Related Problems with General Health

It is neither possible nor helpful to separate all physical problems completely from their psychological components. The two factors are often strongly related. In general practice up to one-fifth of consultations for new episodes of physical illness involve underlying psychological problems, which are revealed when patients are asked the right questions. And of this group, almost three-quarters have diagnosable psychiatric disorders such as anxiety and depression. Surveys of patients in general hospitals show that mental health problems are even more common among people ill enough to have been admitted. Among hospital inpatients psychiatric diagnoses can be made in up to two-fifths.

The relation between physical and psychological problems can work in several ways. Firstly, psychiatric disorders can provoke physical illness in both the short and long term. For example, asthma attacks can be set off by anxiety, and stress seems to contribute to the development of peptic ulcers. Secondly, physical disorders can cause psychiatric symptoms, both as part of the main illness (for instance in thyroid overactivity) and as a later reaction to it. Psychiatrists' general medical training means that they should be able to spot such physical problems.

Lastly, in controversial and puzzling ways sometimes called abnormal illness behaviour, psychological problems can be masked by physical symptoms that have no apparent physical cause. Most people have heard of hypochondriasis, a persistent tendency to worry about health and illness. This is one example of abnormal illness behaviour. Somatization is another example. It means the inability to recognize and deal with anxiety and other stress-related problems, expressing them instead as vague and generalized physical symptoms.

Of course, these medical definitions are inevitably subjective. And they are often unhelpful. After all, what doctor can truthfully say how worried someone should be about their health, or how much psychological stress they are suppressing? None the less, understanding abnormal illness behaviour means that people with hypochondriasis or somatization can be offered psychotherapy, behaviour therapy, and cognitive therapy (see Chapter 2 for details of cognitive therapy).

There are two much stranger, and often more serious examples of abnormal illness behaviour: hysteria and Munchausen's syndrome, in which symptoms and signs of serious physical disease are apparently faked. Munchausen's syndrome is thought to be one of a group of problems called personality disorders and is discussed in more detail on p. 233.

Hysteria is a word that means one thing in common usage and another in medical language. To non-doctors hysteria means overdramatic behaviour which doctors would describe as histrionic. Hysteria as a medical term means an apparent physical problem that has no identifiable physical cause and is thought, instead, to be caused by powerful anxiety that cannot be expressed any other way. The classical example is hysterical blindness which occurs suddenly after seeing something very distressing and resolves again without treatment.

People with hysteria are unaware that the cause is psychological: they do not deliberately fake illness. The whole concept is, of course, shaky because failure to find a physical cause for symptoms does not necessarily mean that there is a psychological cause. Maybe the physical cause is too subtle for examinations and tests to pick up. Indeed, one long-term study showed that at least a third of people diagnosed as hysterical went on to develop genuine neurological diseases after about 10 years.[11] Another third developed depression or schizophrenia, however. Because of this doctors are extremely cautious about using the term hysteria: it is now a very rare diagnosis made only after thorough investigation by specialists.

POST-TRAUMATIC STRESS DISORDER

Survivors of traumatic events like assaults or car crashes commonly develop psychological problems. These problems are called post-traumatic stress disorder when they include vivid and persistent re-experiencing of the traumatic event, phobic avoidance of anything that recalls the event, and a general state of arousal and anxiety (see Box 17). Sufferers re-experience the trauma through intrusive memories, mental images, and dreams. Their lives are hampered by their phobias: car crash survivors may be unable to use any kind of motor transport, for instance. And the anxiety can make them persistently jumpy and irritable and unable to sleep properly. Some sufferers become depressed, often because they feel intensely guilty that they survived while others died, and often because everyday life seems trivial and unimportant in comparison with the awful event.

BOX 17

> **Symptoms of post-traumatic stress disorder**
> - Re-experiencing a traumatic event through intrusive thoughts, mental images, and dreams
> - Avoidance of anything that reminds the sufferer of the trauma
> - Arousal, anxiety, and insomnia

Post-traumatic stress disorder was first named in the USA after it was diagnosed among about a fifth of wounded

Vietnam war veterans. It may well be the same thing as shell shock, which was often diagnosed in soldiers who fought in World War I. During the 1980s post-traumatic stress disorder was found among many survivors of mass disasters and received a lot of attention from the media. Raised awareness of the disorder probably explains why doctors now diagnose it in up to 9% of the general population.[12] More doctors now know to look for the disorder and to ask questions sensitively about past experiences. Raj, who is described here, had post-traumatic stress disorder that his doctor at first did not recognize:

Raj was a 35-year-old shop manager in a large city. Two years previously he had been threatened with a shotgun during an armed robbery by two men who stole the shop's weekly takings. The raid happened on a winter evening. Over the next few months Raj became nervous of working in the evenings, so he changed his shifts. But his nervousness soon affected him at any time of day and he took a week off work.

On returning to the shop after sick leave Raj became extremely anxious. He just could not get the image of the gun out of his head. Whenever he was at work he felt jumpy, and when people walked in the door he felt terrified. Raj vividly imagined that every customer had a gun.

When the symptoms began to occur at home, whenever anyone came to the front door, Raj decided it was time to go to his GP for help. Besides, he had not slept well for months and his wife was worried by his general anxiousness. Raj told his doctor about the insomnia and anxiety. He did not, however, mention the robbery at the shop because he did not think to. Anyway, that happened almost a year earlier.

Raj's doctor checked him physically and asked him what was on his mind. Raj said he was worried about feeling so tired and also said that he had gone off sex. His doctor reassured him that there seemed to be nothing physically wrong, but did some tests to rule out diabetes, and told Raj to come back in a week.

When Raj returned the doctor said that the tests were normal. The doctor then asked more about the insomnia. It was only when Raj mentioned that he had terrible nightmares about the robbery that his doctor began to suspect the right diagnosis. Further questions confirmed Raj's problem and convinced the doctor to refer him to a psychologist for therapy.

Treating Post-Traumatic Stress Disorder
Immediately after the traumatic event medical and social help are often needed more urgently than psychiatric help. Survivors may have physical injuries that need treatment. And if there is financial hardship, perhaps because the family breadwinner has been killed, help from social security and social services may be important.

Psychological symptoms can take at least six months to appear. If they persist for more than a month, the sufferer probably needs professional help. A psychiatrist or other therapist (often a psychologist) will use a mixture of counselling and behaviour therapy. Antidepressant drugs may help too.

Behaviour therapy for this disorder follows the basic principles of exposure therapy, as used for phobias (p. 31). But it is not possible to expose sufferers to the real sources of their fears in the way that agoraphobic people can be taken to the shops: the fears in post-traumatic stress disorder arise from memory. A special kind of exposure must be used, therefore, called image habituation therapy.[13]

During this therapy sufferers are helped to record themselves on audiotape. On the tapes they talk about the traumatic events, describing the recurrent memories that now intrude into their thoughts and dreams. The descriptions can be very brief. Sufferers then listen to each described memory and try to visualize the past event as vividly as possible. This exposure is done gradually and is backed up with methods to deal with the anxiety that occurs during treatment. When the person being treated is used to the technique and can cope with the anxiety that may arise, the tapes can be listened to at home as part of formal 'homework'. Of ten people treated in Vaughan and Tarrier's study six improved considerably after ten homework sessions, two moderately improved, and two did not.

2 DEPRESSION AND MANIC DEPRESSION

Life's Downs and Ups

> Being depressed is like being in a room that needs decorating – you don't know it needs decorating so you can't do anything about it. All you know is a sense of dull misery and bewilderment that you have to stay in such a room.
>
> From *Coping with Anxiety and Depression* by Shirley Trickett[1]

Depression is an overused word. We all have days when we feel fed up and low and some of us describe these feelings as depression. But doctors reserve the term depression for an illness, one that varies in severity but can affect physical health and even threaten life. And sufferers from the illness know all too well the difference between feeling fed up and being really depressed.

Manic depression is something different again: a serious form of depression that recurs through life and that includes episodes of abnormally elevated mood called mania (or its slightly milder form hypomania). Because both the depressive and manic parts of this illness are often accompanied by psychotic symptoms – delusions, hallucinations, and loss of reality sense – psychiatrists sometimes use the term manic depressive psychosis. They also use an even more technical term, bipolar affective disorder, because the illness has two extremes or poles and because it concerns mood, which can also be called affect. Similarly, some psychiatrists use the blanket term affective disorders to cover both depression and manic depression.

In both kinds of affective disorder the mood change is intense and sustained and is often accompanied by alterations in mental, social, and physical functioning. Worrying preoccupations, poor concentration, insomnia, disturbed appetite, and changes in energy level can all occur in both depressive and manic illnesses.

Clearly, what doctors call affective disorders are much more than just moodiness. There are, however, some people who are particularly moody, swinging between cheerfulness and grumpiness from day to day throughout their lives. But it's just how they are: it's part of their personality. Mood swings like these may be hard work, both for the people that have them and for those on the receiving end of them. But they do not usually amount to or lead to illness. A detailed look at depression and manic depression will explain the difference between a moody personality and an affective disorder.

DEPRESSION

Depression is common. Surveys show that up to 15% of the general population complain of some degree of depression at any one time. Around one in five adults suffer depression at some time in their lives. Depression is at least 10 times commoner than manic depression, which is discussed on pp. 84–96. In 1991 government figures estimated that around 2.3 million people in Britain had depression and some 230,000 had manic depression.

Depression can affect anyone, at any age. It is usually most severe, with more disabling symptoms and greater risk to health, when it affects middle-aged and old people. It is diagnosed about twice as often among women as among men. This may mean that women are more likely to become depressed – perhaps because of genes, hormones, childbirth, childcare, lack of paid employment, and women's social roles. On the other hand, the figures may reflect a bias in diagnosing depression – doctors, women's families and partners, and women themselves may all be socially conditioned to recognize depression among women more readily than among men.

To make the figures as accurate as possible doctors try to use standard methods to diagnose depression. But this is not easy, not least because depression's various forms have acquired a confusing array of labels over the years. Perhaps the simplest way to describe depression is to call it mild, moderate, or severe. Indeed, this is what many British psychiatrists do. Some use the American terms – dysthymia for mild or moderate cases and major depression for when symptoms are more severe. Others use more complicated terms to classify depression. These are worth knowing because they may crop up in consultations, in patients' records, and in other books.

One classification defines the problem by its apparent cause: reactive depression occurs in response to a defined stress, while endogenous depression occurs apparently spontaneously and is thought to be caused primarily by a chemical imbalance in the brain. Another method describes the nature of the symptoms: psychotic depression is characterized by delusions, hallucinations, loss of reality, and disturbed behaviour while neurotic depression does not interfere substantially with the brain's functioning.

Lastly, depression can be classified by the pattern it follows. If periods of low mood are interspersed with periods of extreme euphoria (as in manic depression) the illness is described as bipolar, and if the mood change is intermittent but always in the same direction (down) the illness is unipolar. Brief recurrent depression is a new label for frequent episodes that last only a few days but are none the less quite serious and disabling. Seasonal affective disorder is a kind of depression that recurs, but only in winter.

Doctors use labels like these to ensure that they mean the same things when discussing depression. Classifying illnesses can also be useful in choosing treatments; for instance most people with psychotic depression need both antipsychotic and antidepressant medicines. Labels, however, are of little use to most people with depression. Their lives, which are unique and personal and cannot be categorized, get them down. Alison's story is typical:

Alison was a single mother with three young children. She was 28 and had not had paid employment since her second child was born three years earlier. Alison coped well and enjoyed bringing up her children. She had quite a bit of help from her parents, who lived nearby. Her parents, however, had always planned to live on the coast and when her father retired they left.

Alison was surprised at how much she missed them. Gradually, she began to feel low. She lost confidence in her ability to run her family on her own and felt that previously manageable problems like her finances were becoming insurmountable. Increasingly, she blamed herself for her boyfriend leaving her, and felt that she had made a mess of her life. She felt she couldn't do anything right.

Bouts of weeping and worrying exhausted Alison. Extra cigarettes and a few drinks helped her cope, and talking to friends or phoning her parents cheered her up briefly, but she could not shake off the general feeling of depression.

When Alison took her oldest daughter along to the health centre for routine pre-school injections the nurse noticed how tired and fed up she looked. The nurse persuaded Alison to see her GP. The doctor said that the loss of regular contact with her parents had understandably made her feel depressed. She needed support and practical help, however, not tranquillizers or other drugs. The Citizens' Advice Bureau, suggested the doctor, was the place to start.

The staff at the bureau checked all Alison's social security benefits and, on finding that she was entitled to more than she was currently claiming, helped her increase her income. They also advised her to enrol the children at a social services' run day nursery and to get in touch with a counsellor at the local community help centre.

Several sessions with the counsellor helped Alison find better ways of solving problems, revived her self-confidence, and made her feel much more hopeful about the future. Meanwhile the day nursery stimulated and entertained the children, making them much easier to manage. And it allowed Alison to take up part time work, thus boosting her confidence, her social life, and her income.

Six months after her parents moved away, Alison felt more in control of her life.

Signs and Symptoms of Depression

The central symptom of depression is, quite simply, lowered mood. Sufferers describe this as a persistent feeling of sadness, the blues, emptiness, loss, and dread. Some say depression makes everything black – it is like being in a dark hole or tunnel, or having a heavy cloud overhead. Winston Churchill used to call his depression his black dog. And the word melancholy comes from the Greek for black bile, which was once thought to cause depression.

Occasionally, depression is experienced as loss of feeling, as if the emotions are dead. Usually, however, sadness and other unpleasant emotions are keenly felt and only pleasant feelings are hard to find. Sufferers lose interest in their social lives and say that nothing gives them pleasure any more.

Low mood is the main symptom affecting thoughts and feelings in depression, but there are others, mainly affecting thought processes (see Box 1). Calling these symptoms 'psychological' conveys the idea that they concern processes in the mind. It does not necessarily mean that they are not caused by physical disease or disorder within the brain: indeed there is much evidence to suggest that they are often due to chemical imbalances in the brain (see p. 59). But more obviously physical symptoms, affecting the body's whole functioning, can also occur. When they do, they are usually a sign of severe depression.

BOX 1	**Psychological symptoms that may occur in depression**
	Low mood
	Depressive thoughts
	worries
	poor self-image, low self-confidence, self-blame and guilt
	negative thoughts about the world and the future
	hopelessness
	Suicidal thoughts
	Psychotic symptoms
	hallucinations
	delusions

Psychological Symptoms

DEPRESSIVE THOUGHTS

Thought processes are usually affected by depression. Probably the commonest kinds of disturbance are poor concentration and a tendency to worry a lot ('I kept on losing track of things and going back to worrying'). Indeed, depression often overlaps with another common mental health problem; anxiety (see Chapter 1 for more information about anxiety and its associated symptoms). Depressive worries, which psychiatrists sometimes call ruminations, are usually about personal problems and challenges that would normally be manageable. As well as having personal worries, depressed people sometimes become oversensitive to sad or gloomy events that do not directly impinge on them, for example disasters and deaths heard about through the media ('I couldn't watch a sad film without crying myself').

Underlying the tendency to worry in depression there are often more general preoccupations. Depressed people may stop liking themselves, lose confidence in themselves, blame themselves for everything, and feel generally guilty ('I feel such a burden to everybody'). Feelings like these can make sufferers think about themselves, the world, and the future in a pervasively negative way. Some theorists believe that negative thoughts actually precede the onset of depression in certain people. Such people are intrinsically more pessimistic and self-critical than others and are especially prone to getting depressed when faced with stressful events, according to one explanation of depression, which is called cognitive theory (see pp. 63–4).

In depression, negative feelings about the future range from doubt and anxiety through to complete lack of hope. Hopelessness suggests real despondency, close to rock bottom. It underlies many suicidal thoughts.

SUICIDAL THOUGHTS
Thoughts of self-harm or suicide are common in depression. They vary in intensity from fleeting vague thoughts, for example that not waking up one morning would be a relief, to strong and clear ideas about preparing for and carrying out a viable suicide plan.

About 15% of people who become depressed at some time during their lives eventually kill themselves. Depression is not the only cause of suicide; it accounts for about half of all cases each year in Britain. Because suicide is a complex subject and because it has many causes, it has its own chapter in this book (see pp. 235–57). The importance of suicide as a major public health problem has not escaped the government, either. They have set targets for health and local authorities to reduce the overall suicide rate by at least 15% by the year 2000 and to reduce the rate among mentally ill people by a third in the same period.

Suicide due to depression can be prevented. The government and NHS can prevent suicide by helping GPs to recognize and treat depression more effectively; psychiatric staff can prevent it by improving support and supervision of suicidal patients; and confidantes (families, friends, therapists and counsellors, the Samaritans) can prevent it by being there when needed. Chapter 8 gives more detailed advice on dealing with suicidal feelings. One of the keys to this is to understand how suicidal feelings develop. Brian's story shows how this can happen:

Brian was a 40-year-old married man who had been off sick for three weeks from his job as a salesman in a DIY store. Over the past year he had been under mounting pressure to increase sales, on which much of his income depended. He had worked well but he saw himself as a failure, perhaps because he was a bit of a perfectionist. To make matters worse, the long working hours and his continual tiredness were putting a strain on his marriage.

Brian felt exhausted and found everything an effort. Over the past six months he had lost his appetite and more than a stone in weight. He was waking at 5 o'clock most mornings, turning over his problems in his mind and dreading the day. He had lost interest in most things, including sex.

When Brian went off sick things got worse. Without the daily distraction of work he felt desperately low. He even cried at times, something he had not done since his father died 10 years earlier. His wife tried in vain to reassure him. She persuaded him to go to their GP, who realized that Brian was depressed and started him on a course of antidepressant tablets.

Brian took the tablets reluctantly for a couple of days. But he was not convinced that they could help him. He felt overwhelmed by feelings of worthlessness and fears that he was never going to cope with his workload. Deciding that he was hopeless, and an unacceptable burden to his family, he took all his tablets in one go.

His wife came home from work early and found him alive but unconscious. He was admitted to hospital and, once he had recovered from the physical effects of the overdose, he was transferred to a psychiatric unit.

Very occasionally someone who is severely depressed commits suicide and homicide at the same time, perhaps killing a partner or child. Underlying this is an overwhelming and unrealistic hopelessness about the future for everyone. Thus, the depressed person can see murder as a merciful release for his or her nearest and dearest. But this is very rare, and depressed people are not usually dangerous to anyone else.

PSYCHOTIC SYMPTOMS

Depression can develop as a psychosis, which means that the sufferer loses touch with reality and experiences very abnormal symptoms such as hallucinations and delusions. Distinguishing psychotic depression from schizophrenia can be difficult, particularly if the person has not been ill before and there is no previous pattern to compare with. The main difference is that, in depression, clear symptoms of low mood are usually present from the outset. Another clue is that the hallucinations and delusions usually have a particularly gloomy or self-blaming content.

Depressive hallucinations tend to reinforce the low mood and negative thoughts. Sufferers feeling guilty and worthless may hear one or more insulting or highly critical voices ('There's no hope', 'You have to die now'). Depressive delusions also tend to fit with the mood: for instance, sufferers wrongly become convinced that they have caused catastrophes, or have committed great sins and crimes ('I knew I had caused the famine in Ethiopia'). More strangely, and more rarely, they may believe that part of the body has stopped working or even died, despite clear evidence to the contrary ('My bowels have completely blocked up with cancer'). Extremely negative delusions of this type are called nihilistic (after the philosophical concept of nihilism: belief in nothing). Catherine, described below, had delusions like this.

> Catherine had a long history of recurrent depression which started after the birth of her son 50 years earlier. Now, aged 73 and recently widowed, she was ill again. Her grief over her husband's death wasn't lessening,

even though he had been dead for nearly nine months. Catherine was withdrawing into herself, avoiding contact with other people in the village and almost becoming a recluse. She didn't care about herself or how she looked any more. She was getting very thin.

Eventually, when no one had seen her for days and she was not answering the door or telephone, a worried neighbour broke in to her house. Catherine was in bed, looking emaciated and dehydrated. Her hands were very cold. She was uncommunicative, just staring into space.

Catherine's doctor came and got her into hospital. With fluids by intravenous drip and antibiotics for a chest infection Catherine became stronger physically within a couple of days. But she remained withdrawn and refused to eat anything, only taking sips of water after great persuasion. Little by little, she confided in one nurse and explained why she had neglected herself so much.

Catherine believed that her insides were blocked up by some disease and that she was about to die. She deserved to die, she said, because she hadn't done enough for her husband during his last illness. Death would be a welcome release because she had huge debts and no money. By now, she said, her house would have been taken away because of rent arrears.

None of these ideas was true: they were depressive delusions that she firmly believed. Medical examinations and tests showed Catherine's insides to be fine. Her son said that she was financially secure, that the house had been mortgaged and paid off long ago, and that she had looked after his father tirelessly. But Catherine could not be reassured and still refused to eat. She agreed, however, to be moved over to the psychiatric unit.

Catherine had delusions that made her too scared to eat. But she may also have had a physical loss of appetite, particularly in the early stages of her depression. Poor appetite and weight loss are two of the commonest physical symptoms of depression.

Physical Symptoms in Depression

As if feeling psychologically low wasn't enough, depression can cause a whole range of physical problems (see Box 2). Bouts of depression that include symptoms like these tend to be longer lasting and more serious than those with only psychological symptoms. And they usually respond much more readily to physical treatments such as antidepressants and electric shock treatment (electroconvulsive therapy or ECT).

Depression usually makes people feel generally unwell. They feel tired, unable to muster energy or enthusiasm for anything, unable to concentrate, and not interested in food or sex ('I haven't got any motivation for anything. Everything is too much of an effort'). This malaise can lead to weight loss, constipation, and insomnia. The insomnia classically occurs in the early hours of the morning. The sufferer wakes at 4 or 5 o'clock then dozes fitfully or lies awake till morning, with repetitive worries churning round the mind like clothes in a washing machine ('I wake up and it's there immediately – worry, tension, all the feelings'). Exhaustion and a feeling of pessimism or dread about the day ahead then make getting up very hard. Even when sleep is not affected, depressed people tend to feel lowest in the mornings.

Other physical symptoms are less common but tend to be more disabling. Severe depression can temporarily slow down the whole mind and body, causing a problem that doctors call psychomotor retardation. Some people say this feels like wading through syrup, with every thought and action requiring a huge effort. This slowing may be obvious, causing quiet, halting, and monotonous speech and sluggish movements. Among elderly people the converse, agitation, is fairly common in depression. Mental confusion – causing muddled thinking, poor memory, and disorientation – can also complicate severe depression among elderly sufferers. This may be so marked and persistent that people think the old person has developed dementia, indeed, this kind of depression is sometimes called pseudodementia.

BOX 2

Physical symptoms that may occur in depression

Loss of energy

Loss of appetite and weight, constipation

Going off sex

Insomnia

Disturbed body rhythm

    daily variation – feeling worst in mornings

    seasonal variation – becoming depressed in winter

Poor concentration

Slowing of actions and thoughts

Agitation   } particularly among
Mental confusion } elderly sufferers

Causes of Depression

Most people trying to understand why they became depressed tend to look first at recent events for explanations. Many find that their depressions start as extensions of unhappiness. But not everyone who has to deal with sad feelings gets depressed: some people seem intrinsically at greater risk than others. Research on depression supports this idea and suggests that events early in life increase the risk, while later events act as triggering or precipitating factors. These factors are summarized in Box 3.

BOX 3   **Probable causes of depression**

Risk factors
- Inheritance
- Brain abnormalities
- Vulnerability factors

Precipitating factors
- Psychological triggers

Stress

Loss and bereavement

Depressive thinking
- Physical triggers

Some physical illnesses

Childbirth

Menstrual cycle

Lack of daylight

Virus infections

Alcohol and drug misuse

Risk Factors in Depression

Inheritance
As with any condition, whether illness or financial wealth, the fact that depression runs in families does not prove genetic inheritance. And there is little evidence that mild forms of depression, which comprise the majority, are caused by genetic problems as opposed to social and emotional factors. This may be because the many social and emotional explanations for mild depression cloud the picture and because less research has been done on the earlier causes.

Research on the causes of severe depression does suggest a genetic component (the principles of genetic studies are explained in detail in the chapter on schizophrenia). In brief, identical twins of depressed people have a 70% chance of developing depression themselves compared with a 13% chance for non-identical twins (who are genetically no closer than ordinary siblings) and a 10–15% chance for other close relatives. Thus, relatives whose genes are most similar to depressed people are also likely to develop depression.

Genetics might also play a role in women's tendency to become depressed. Gender is carried by the sex chromosomes, which comprise one of the 23 pairs of gene packages in each human being. Women have two X chromosomes (so called because they are cross-shaped when seen under a microscope), men have one X and one Y. Several illnesses and physical abnormalities are known to affect men and women differently because of defects in the sex chromosomes: depression could, conceivably, be partly explained by a defect that has not yet been discovered.

Brain Abnormalities
Certain chemicals in the brain go haywire during some attacks of depression, particularly in the more severe types with marked physical symptoms. Research has shown decreased levels of two chemicals during such attacks; in particular, serotonin (also known as 5HT) and noradrenaline. These are neurotransmitters, chemicals which carry messages across the gaps between the brain's nerves. When their supply is depleted the wrong messages are sent, and depressive symptoms could be one kind of faulty response to this. Advances in treatment support this theory: drugs which are known to increase the brain levels of serotonin and noradrenaline are effective antidepressants.

What causes these chemical abnormalities is not yet clear. Some researchers think that the imbalance in brain chemistry is genetic, and that this is how depression is inherited. Others think that unhappiness and sadness trigger the chemical imbalances in otherwise normal brains. After all, psychological factors are known to affect other brain functions – for example, worrying about an unwanted pregnancy can upset the brain's pituitary gland and thereby delay an expected period.

Vulnerability Factors
Extensive research on women in London during the 1970s found that certain social and emotional factors made them particularly prone to depression. Women were at considerable risk of getting depressed if they lacked someone to confide in, had no employment outside the home, had more than three children under 14, and had lost their mothers by death or long-term separation during childhood.[2] Later research has had conflicting results, but most has given some support to Brown and Harris's theory.

Another kind of event that can make girls vulnerable to depression and other mental health problems in later life is physical or sexual abuse. Surveys suggest that up to a half of all women in psychiatric wards and outpatient clinics have had some kind of unwanted sexual attention during childhood or early adolescence. Similar surveys of adult women in the general population suggest that far fewer, around 15–20%, have had such experiences. Critics say that women with mental health problems may not have reliable memories of early experiences and say that it is hard, anyway, to get honest answers to personal and distressing questions about sex. But recent surveys[3] using tried and tested questionnaires and interview techniques have consistently shown a link between childhood sexual abuse and later mental illness.

Precipitating Factors
In the same way that both psychological and physical factors seem to increase the risk of getting depression, both kinds of factor can trigger or precipitate bouts.

Psychological Triggers for Depression

STRESS

Like anxiety, depression can arise from chronic and overwhelming stresses in life. Brian, described earlier, became depressed when pressures at work became hard to bear. He lost confidence in his ability to cope and eventually lost confidence in himself altogether. Why Brian should have become depressed, rather than anxious, is not clear. He probably had a mixture of reasons to become depressed, including a strong and unresolved sense of loss following his father's death.

LOSS AND BEREAVEMENT

Many of the psychological stresses that lead to depression can be summed up under the concept of loss. The type of loss may be obvious – loss of a loved one through death or separation, failure of a business, being made redundant. But the loss may be more subtle – loss of self-esteem in a destructive relationship, loss of ability and health because of physical illness, infertility, miscarriage, or loss of hopes for the future. For most of us, however, bereavement due to a loved one's death is the most devastating form of loss.

Extensive research shows that most people who recover normally after bereavement have symptoms in the first year that would, at other times, suggest mental illness, particularly depression. Most of this research has been performed by the British psychiatrist Colin Murray Parkes, who has identified normal grieving as a three-stage process (see Box 4 for summary).

BOX 4 | **Normal Grieving**

There are three phases:

1. Numbness – lasting about a week, although some feelings of disbelief may persist for several months

> 2. Mourning – acutely for up to three months, with strong feelings of sadness, guilt, and anger; restlessness; and sometimes with hallucinations. Resolves between 3–6 months after the death
> 3. Acceptance – from 6 months onwards

The first experience of grief is usually a state of shock. For up to a week, while organizing the funeral, the bereaved person may feel numb and feel that nothing, not even the death, is real. Other people think that he or she is taking it all remarkably well.

The second stage of grieving starts abruptly, after a week or two, with an acute and intensely painful sense of loss. The bereaved person feels wretched and desperate and soon becomes exhausted by crying, insomnia, poor concentration, and loss of appetite. About a third of bereaved people have strong guilty feelings that they did not do enough for the person who died, and about a fifth feel intense anger towards doctors, other professionals, and even God, for failing to prevent the death.

This phase of mourning is just like depression in about half of all bereaved people. Anxiety commonly occurs too, associated with restlessness and an urge to search for the dead person, as if he or she has merely gone away somewhere.

During this phase of mourning symptoms can occur that are sufficiently strange to suggest mental illness, but are actually transient and solely caused by intense grief. Brief hallucinations of the dead person may occur: about one in ten of recently bereaved people see or hear their dead relatives and friends while awake. Intrusive thoughts and disturbing dreams may also add to the distress. John Milton described this well in the poem *On His Dead Wife*, about a man's dream of his dead wife:

> Methought I saw my late espousèd Saint
> Brought to me like *Alcestis* from the grave,

Whom *Jove*'s great Son to her glad Husband gave,
  Rescu'd from death by force though pale and faint.
Mine as whom washed from spot of child-bed taint,
  Purification in the old Law did save,
  And such, as yet once more I trust to have
Full sight of her in Heaven without restraint,
Came vested all in white, pure as her mind:
  Her face was vail'd, yet to my fancied sight
  Love, sweetness, goodness, in her person shin'd
So clear, as in no face with more delight.
  But O as to embrace me she enclin'd,
  I wak'd, she fled, and day brought back my night.

Despite intense experiences like these, most bereaved people manage to carry on with their normal routines and jobs. Most of those seeking medical help can be reassured that all of this is normal and that, by six months, the symptoms will usually ease off considerably. From then on the bereaved person learns how to build a new life and, to some extent, a new identity. But some bereavement reactions have devastating effects that interrupt daily life completely and some persist for many months, even years. The bereaved person may develop any clear-cut and full-blown psychiatric illness, but depression is the commonest response. If this is associated with suicidal feelings or other life-threatening symptoms such as complete refusal to eat, admission to hospital will probably be necessary.

DEPRESSIVE THINKING

The concept that certain patterns of thinking precede and cause depression has already been mentioned on pp. 51–2. Since the late 1970s theorists led by Aaron T. Beck, an American professor of psychiatry, have been developing the cognitive theory as an explanation of many psychological problems, particularly depression. Beck says that some people are unduly negative about themselves, the world, and the future and that their pessimistic thoughts (or, more technically, cognitions) make them at risk of depression.

Beck says that such people have three problems with their thinking. Firstly, they set high and unrealistic conditions for their happiness ('I'll only be happy if I'm successful in everything I do', 'My self-worth depends entirely on what others think of me'). Secondly, they take things too personally ('He's not interested in me so I must be unattractive to all men', 'I can't get promotion so I'm an all-round failure'). And, lastly, their negative thoughts occur spontaneously and intrusively (or, as Beck says, they get 'automatic' negative thoughts that are hard to stop). These three problems of thinking lead into and perpetuate depression, according to cognitive theory.

Cognitive theory is gaining more and more support because cognitive therapy, the treatment that undoes these ways of thinking, is proving to be an effective cure for mild and moderate depression (see p. 74).

Physical Triggers for Depression
Many physical illnesses can trigger depression. These include viral infections, hormonal conditions such as thyroid disease, neurological disease such as multiple sclerosis and epilepsy, and cancer. In women, depression has been linked to the menstrual cycle, the menopause, and childbirth. Of all these physical triggers, childbirth is the most common and clear cut.

CHILDBIRTH
In the first year after childbirth women are five times more likely to suffer psychiatric problems than at other times of life, and in the first three months the risk is sixteen times greater than normal. Although most of these problems are relatively mild and do not seriously interfere with the mother's life or ability to care for her baby, they are sufficiently common to warrant detailed description.

More than half of all mothers experience transient baby blues in the first week after childbirth. These episodes of tearfulness, general gloominess, and irritability typically follow a couple of days of mostly good feelings with elation and excitement. The blues usually start suddenly on or around the fourth day, often coinciding with the return home from hospital. By definition these transient mood changes clear up completely and quickly – usually by the end of the first week – and need nothing more than support and understanding from those nearby.

The consistent and clear pattern of the blues suggests a single cause, most probably a physical one related to the huge hormonal changes that occur around the time of childbirth and the start of breastfeeding. And in 1994, after years of trying in vain because hormone levels are technically difficult to measure, researchers showed that the baby blues are probably linked to a steep drop in progesterone levels in the body.[4]

However, the researchers called the link between the blues and the hormones only 'weak and modest', and the physical changes may be only part of the story. The powerful psychological changes that occur within mothers and their families after birth (particularly after the first, which is most frequently followed by the blues) may be more than enough to explain what happens. As consultant psychotherapist Jane Price says in her book *Motherhood – What it does to your mind*:

> Motherhood can be the best or worst emotional experience of a woman's life . . . Most girls grow up believing that they will have children and that this will give them credibility as women as well as providing a fundamental form of fulfilment. The facts that it will also make them emotionally vulnerable, place severe practical limits around their lives, and require that they rapidly achieve heights of adult responsibility that few other situations in life demand are often the hidden cost of the experience.[5]

Dr Price goes on to explain that our society is very bad at acknowledging the negative effects of motherhood:

> It is a fascinating part of our cultural mythology that motherhood is given such a rosy write-up everywhere and that the other, much blacker, side of the bargain is hardly mentioned . . . To speak against the myths of

motherhood risks the individual woman being branded a bad mother, a fate most women would do much to avoid. Even amongst women there is a degree of silence about the reality of mothering . . .[6]

When mothers get the baby blues they feel fed up but do not usually feel ill. But the postnatal depression that follows 15–20% of pregnancies can cause definite and persistent symptoms, just like those that occur in depressive illnesses at other times of life. The scale of postnatal depression tends to diminish over time, with the severest forms occurring soonest after the birth and the mildest last. Vague forms of depression, often with anxiety and other relatively mild psychiatric symptoms, typically start between three months and a year postnatally. This delay may be because the celebration, attention, and support that families, friends, and health professionals give new mothers keep them going in the first three months or so.

Most women with depression serious enough to need treatment develop symptoms two to four weeks after the birth. But about a quarter of serious cases start abruptly within the first two weeks.

About a third of these early severe postnatal psychiatric illnesses are accounted for by postnatal psychosis, with disturbed behaviour and thinking and hallucinations and delusions. Some of these psychoses are accompanied by mania rather than depression, and some do not have very marked mood changes but resemble attacks of schizophrenia.

For many years scientific researchers have tried to explain all these postnatal illnesses by looking for a physical cause such as hormonal change. But, apart from the probable hormonal link to the baby blues, no clear biological explanation has been found. Medical and social researchers, however, have noticed certain factors that are commonly associated with, and seem to increase the risk of developing, postnatal psychiatric problems (see Box 5).

BOX 5

Factors that increase the risk of developing postnatal psychiatric illness

Problems before pregnancy

- postnatal psychiatric illness in the past
- death of a previous baby
- any severe mental illness in the past, or in the family
- unusual age for pregnancy – mother a teenager or over 35
- single parenthood
- serious financial problems and poverty

Problems during pregnancy

- strong mixed feelings about having the baby
- abortion considered
- scares about baby's health, e.g. growth rate queried by doctors
- admission to antenatal ward for more than a week
- worrying events in last three months of pregnancy, e.g. moving house
- difficult labour, e.g. needing caesarean operation

Problems after the birth

- ill baby, especially if taken immediately to intensive care
- ill mother, e.g. with haemorrhage
- feelings of loss of independence, financial security, status especially if not returning to previous job

- shock and disappointment if expectations of motherhood were unrealistic and are not met
- social isolation
- lack of emotional support

THE MENSTRUAL CYCLE

The physical stresses of menstruation and the menopause vary from woman to woman and so do the psychological stresses. Up to three-quarters of all women may become irritable, snappy, and low premenstrually, with breast tenderness and bloating. But relatively few feel bad enough to seek medical help. If the physical symptoms start more than a day or two (and sometimes as long as a fortnight) before each period they are considered by many doctors to be abnormal, amounting to premenstrual syndrome. No clear link has been found between hormone fluctuations and mood fluctuations. Some women complaining of depression or anxiety premenstrually have symptoms all month, with only slight exacerbations before their periods.

The menopause is another time when women may feel depressed and irritable, with poor concentration. But researchers who have conducted extensive surveys of women in Britain, the United States, Canada and Sweden say that, although some women do get depressed around the menopause, the numbers are no greater than at other times of life.[7]

Most psychiatrists believe that social and emotional changes are more important than biology in explaining postmenopausal depression.[8] Common stresses for women aged 40–50 include sadness at loss of fertility and at children leaving home, and fears about ageing – all of which can cause a feeling of uselessness that is sometimes called the redundancy syndrome.

Medical research has not, therefore, established whether the reproductive cycle substantially increases women's vulnerability to psychiatric illness, even though the possibility makes sense. Many psychiatrists believe that women who complain of psychological symptoms before periods and around the time of the menopause have other underlying problems that make them generally vulnerable. This tendency to apply a general label of vulnerability rather than to use a specific physical explanation could be seen as discriminatory and dismissive, and as a reflection of the fact that, until recently, most doctors and medical researchers were men. But even female psychiatrists who specialize in women's problems agree that there are few grounds to blame hormones for everything. Pamela Ashurst and Zaida Hall say in their book *Understanding Women in Distress*:

> Research evidence is conflicting, but it seems likely that menopausal depression is, like postnatal depression, multifactorial in origin. There are undoubtedly hormonal changes and alterations in body rhythm, but most women manage to survive this without psychological disturbance.[9]

LACK OF DAYLIGHT

Many of us find bright sunny days more cheering than dark gloomy days. But some people seem particularly sensitive to daylight, and develop persistent and marked depression as the days shorten with the onset of winter. This winter depression or seasonal affective disorder may be caused by an imbalance of the hormone melatonin. Melatonin is released by the brain's pineal gland during darkness and suppressed during daylight. It is thought to regulate the body's time clock and to cause sleepiness at night. It may also cause depression in some people; a theory that is supported by treatment trials showing that regular exposure to intense light can banish seasonal affective disorder. Treatment using melatonin is still in the experimental stages.

VIRUS INFECTIONS

Depression sometimes occurs soon after an acute viral infection, for instance flu, glandular fever, hepatitis, or shingles. Whether the depression is triggered by some physical mechanism or is a psychological response to being laid up is not clear. Whatever the exact cause, postviral depression is usually fairly mild, clearing up within a few weeks.

Chronic fatigue syndrome or ME (myalgic encephalomyelitis) is a long-term problem of lethargy, tiredness, and muscle aching on exertion. It is three times commoner among women than men and usually starts between ages 30 and 40. Some people believe the syndrome is caused by persistent viral infection, in particular with the Epstein-Barr virus that causes glandular fever and the Coxsackie virus that causes infections of the heart muscle. But viruses are found in only a few sufferers from chronic fatigue syndrome whereas depression (often an unusual kind without the feelings of guilt and unworthiness that are common in depression) is found in three-quarters. And scientific tests on sufferers' muscles shows no physical explanation for the feeling of fatigue. The most successful treatments so far have been programmes of gradually increasing exercise and courses of antidepressants.

Lack of a known physical cause for the syndrome does not mean, however, that the fatigue is not real. It suggests simply that the fatigue is sensed centrally, in the brain, rather than in the muscles. As Professor P. K. Thomas of the Royal Free Hospital in London says:

> The fatigue that patients with the chronic fatigue syndrome experience is an exceedingly discomforting symptom and must have a neural correlate. So far the physiology of central fatigue is largely unexplored . . . Possibly the setting of the neural mechanisms responsible for this sensation is altered in patients with the chronic fatigue syndrome and depression, in the same way that in anorexia nervosa the body image may be altered.[10]

ALCOHOL AND DRUG MISUSE

People with alcohol and drug problems may get severely depressed and even attempt suicide. Indeed, alcohol and drug misuse, which are discussed in detail in Chapter 5, account for about one in four suicides each year in Britain.

Treatments for Depression

Most people with depression never seek professional help. They wait for it to pass naturally or find ways to combat it. For those who know what has been getting them down, maybe a difficult relationship or a stressful situation, efforts to overcome or remove the cause are often successful. And confiding in friends and relatives can make a huge difference – the old saying that a problem shared is a problem halved is often true.

But many people look for outside help in getting through depression. Some find self-help groups and books useful (see Box 6 for examples). Others go to their GPs or community mental health centres for professional help and treatment.

BOX 6 | **Self-Help for Depression**

Two national organizations offer advice specifically on depression, as well as support to sufferers and their relatives:

Fellowship of Depressives Anonymous

Depressives Associated

Britain's Royal College of Psychiatrists provides educational information on depression as part of its Defeat Depression campaign. The five-year campaign was started in January 1992 to raise public awareness about depression, and to explain that depression is common, recognizable, and treatable.

The following books may help too:

Depression and its Treatment by John Hinton (Family Doctor Publications, British Medical Association, 1986)

Coping with Anxiety and Depression by Shirley Trickett (Sheldon Press, 1989)

Postnatal Depression by Vivienne Welburn (Fontana, 1980)

By and large, treatments and the settings in which they are given vary according to the severity. Most people with depression do best at home where they are on familiar territory and have the support of family and friends. All the professional help may come from the GP. Sometimes more help is needed and, in well-run local health services, GPs can call on other community services such as community psychiatric nursing.

Community nurses offer psychological support to sufferers and their families, monitor the severity of symptoms, and can bring in other services like day centres. They can also assess the need for and provide specific programmes of treatment, for instance when a depressed person also has agoraphobia. Increasingly, this role is being extended to other members of community mental health teams such as occupational therapists and social workers.

GPs and other community staff call on psychiatrists to help when patients are not recovering as expected and when depression is too severe to manage at home. Even if a sufferer has to see a psychiatrist, this does not mean having to go to hospital. Psychiatrists see most depressed people in outpatient clinics, GPs' surgeries or, sometimes, in the patients' own homes.

The commonest reasons for admission to hospital are inability to cope at home and suicide risk. Ideally, hospitals offer a safe environment that relieves depressed people of their routine burdens and responsibilities, allows them to concentrate on getting better, and can provide intensive treatment.

Treatments for depression include psychological, practical, and physical measures. There are also some specialized approaches, for example for postnatal and postmenopausal depression.

Psychological and Practical Treatments for Depression

COUNSELLING AND PSYCHOTHERAPY
Counselling is a professional extension of the help that friends and family can provide, and it is probably helpful in all kinds of depression. Many general practices now employ counsel-

lors to see, among others, people with depression. And most medical and nursing staff in general practice and hospital settings use counselling skills in their daily work. The general principles of counselling and psychotherapy, the 'talking cures', have already been described in the Introduction.

When depression is part of a complicated reaction to bereavement special counselling can be used to overcome grief (see Box 7). For other sources of expert advice and information on bereavement see Box 8. The symptoms of normal grieving usually last 6–12 months, although it can take years to feel completely happy again. Feelings of grief may surge back briefly at certain times – for example at Christmas, birthdays, and anniversaries. Psychiatric problems arising from abnormal grieving have variable prognoses, depending on the type of problem and on the usual factors that affect recovery. Follow up of people who have special bereavement counselling and those who contact self-help groups shows that both forms of support can be very effective.

BOX 7	**Principles of bereavement counselling**
	1. Help to acknowledge the loss – talk about when and how it happened, running through the details repeatedly
	2. Help to experience the pain – encourage expression of sadness, despair, anger and guilt
	3. Identify ways of coping and sources of support – who else can help
	4. Help to build a new life without the dead person – identify major decisions to be made and use the list as a focus for action
	5. Help to let go of the dead person – challenge feelings of long-term 'duty' to the deceased and encourage new friendships and relationships. Challenge guilty feelings that letting go is wrong

BOX 8

Self-Help for Bereavement

You can contact the following organizations for help:

- CRUSE-Bereavement Care
- Lesbian and Gay Bereavement Project
- Terrence Higgins Trust
- Compassionate Friends
- Foundation for the Study of Infant Deaths
- The Stillbirth and Neonatal Death Association (SANDS)
- The Cot Death Society
- The Miscarriage Association

These books may also help:
On Death and Dying by Elizabeth Kubler-Ross (Tavistock 1969)

Bereavement: Studies of Grief in Adult Life by Colin M. Parkes (Penguin Books, 1987)

COGNITIVE THERAPY

The theory that underlies this treatment is explained on pp. 63–4. In essence cognitive therapy retrains the mind to question and banish depressive thoughts, change emotional responses, and change behaviour.

People offered a course of cognitive therapy will see a trained therapist, probably a psychologist or community nurse, for 10–20 sessions. In the first session the therapist will explain the theory and the treatment, agree on a structure for the whole course, and start to identify the depressive ways of thinking. Later the depressed person will be shown how to recognize unduly and unrealistically negative thoughts and record them in a special diary. Then he or she will be shown how to test these thoughts against reality.

For example, a thought such as 'I wasn't promoted because I'm useless' would be written down in the diary. The therapist would talk through what was underlying this thought and show the depressed person how to add an alternative and much more realistic explanation next to that entry in the diary. Lack of promotion, for instance, could also be due to factors in work experience, which the person could change and improve. With a mixture of pen and paper tasks, role playing, and counselling, the depressed person will learn to think more positively.

A large body of research has shown that cognitive therapy works in depression. It is quick, taking 10–30 hours in all; it is safe; and it is relatively cheap. And it is particularly useful for people who do not want to take antidepressants. Not surprisingly, cognitive therapy is becoming more widely available in the NHS.

Physical Treatments for Depression

ANTIDEPRESSANTS
Antidepressants include a wide range of different drugs (see Box 9) whose main common feature is the ability to relieve depressed mood. They are quite distinct from the tranquillizers like diazepam (trade name Valium) and are not addictive.

All the antidepressants available currently are more or less equally effective. In studies where patients agree to take either antidepressants or identical dummy 'placebo' pills, without knowing which they are given, at least two-thirds of those who get antidepressants feel much better within three months. Fewer than one-third of those on the inactive placebos recover naturally in the same period. Of course this method, which allows researchers to separate out the possible psychological effect of being given a pill of any description from the real effect of taking antidepressants, is explained to the patients before they take part.

BOX 9   **Types of antidepressant**

Tricyclics

amitriptyiline (Tryptizol)

imipramine (Tofranil)

clomipramine (Anafranil)

dothiepin (Prothiaden)

lofepramine (Gamanil)

Monoamine oxidase inhibitors (MAOIs)

phenelzine (Nardil)

isocarboxazid (Marplan)

tranylcypromine (Parnate)

Selective serotonin reuptake inhibitors (SSRIs)

fluoxetine (Prozac)

fluvoxamine (Faverin)

sertraline (Lustral)

paroxetine (Seroxat)

The most widely prescribed type of antidepressants are the tricyclics, so called because their molecular structure includes three rings. The other commonly used types are named after the actions they have on chemicals in the brain: the specific serotonin reuptake inhibitors (shortened, thankfully, to SSRIs) and the monoamine oxidase inhibitors (MAOIs). All types of antidepressant work in similar ways. But, because the few differences between them are important, it is worth describing the types in some detail.

Tricyclic antidepressants have been used widely since the late 1950s and have cured depression in millions of people. But, initially, they can add to the misery of depression by causing unpleasant side effects. These include sedation, dry mouth, excessive sweating, constipation, urinary problems (particularly in older men with enlarged prostate glands), and impotence (inability to get an erection). These side effects do not affect everybody equally and often decrease considerably or completely after the first week of treatment, leaving only slight dryness of the mouth. Proper warnings about side effects makes them much less alarming and encourages sufferers to persevere with treatment. Up to half of all people prescribed tricyclics, however, cannot tolerate the side effects and stop treatment before their depression is properly treated. More seriously, tricyclics can upset the heart rhythm in susceptible people and should seldom be given in the presence of heart disease.

The SSRIs are relatively new, coming into wide use in the late 1980s. They have had widespread publicity because some doctors in the US claim (without supporting evidence from research and amid much scepticism from other psychiatrists) that SSRIs, particularly Prozac (fluoxetine), can revitalize and cheer up people who are not even depressed. Few, if any doctors in Britain would prescribe antidepressants to healthy people on the basis of current knowledge. But many are prescribing SSRIs to people with depression because the drugs increase the levels in the brain of the chemical messenger serotonin or 5HT, which is thought to be depleted in depression. Indeed, the SSRIs are as effective as tricyclics and, although they can cause nausea and excessive sweating at first, they generally have fewer side effects. Their main disadvantage, however, is that they cost 100 times more than the most commonly used tricyclic, amitriptyline – over £30 compared with just 34 pence for a month's treatment at 1992 prices.[11] Financial considerations may seem petty. But, given the facts that funding for the NHS cannot be bottomless and that British GPs diagnose depression in around 2 million people a year, it is reasonable to expect expensive treatments to be much better than cheap ones. And SSRIs are not more effective than tricyclics. On the other hand, they are more acceptable to many patients and they cause fewer dropouts from treatment – up to a quarter rather than a half. The money saved by completed, successful treatment, may outweigh the prescribing costs.

The last group of antidepressants, the MAOIs, have been in use since the late 1950s. They were developed after a chance observation that patients with tuberculosis cheered up when given an antibiotic that happened to affect the levels of monoamine neurotransmitters in the brain. The MAOIs are stimulants, rather than sedatives, and are particularly helpful for people who are physically and mentally sluggish because of depression. They work well but have one big disadvantage that limits their safety and acceptability: a dangerous interaction with certain foods and other drugs. If taken with the foods and drugs shown in Box 10 (which often contain high levels of a substance called tyramine) MAOIs can cause a sudden and very dangerous increase in blood pressure. People taking them have to carry round an information card explaining the risk and listing the things to avoid. Because of this risk MAOIs are not used much now, except when other treatments have failed. A new MAOI, moclobemide, which does not interact with tyramine to cause high blood pressure, is now available.

BOX 10 **Foods and drugs that must not be taken with MAOIs**

- Cheese, pickled herrings, broad bean pods
- Bovril, Oxo, Marmite and any other meat or yeast extract
- Offal, game, and any meat or fish that may be going off
- Alcohol, particularly Chianti wine
- Any drug taken without consulting a doctor or pharmacist who knows you're on an MAOI (do not even take nose drops, inhalations, suppositories, cold cures, cough medicines, pain killers, laxatives, or tonics)

In general, antidepressants work by restoring the balance of chemicals in the brain. Although they may do this partly by replacing depleted chemicals, this does not explain how they produce a lasting cure or why they have the peculiar feature of taking two to four weeks to start working. The current idea is that antidepressants reinstate normal function by altering the way chemical receptors work in the brain.

Improved sleep and a decrease in anxiety are usually the first signs of improvement, particularly among people taking the more sedative tricyclic drugs. Improvement in other symptoms follows, with the mood starting to lift after about two weeks of treatment. Some people suddenly feel brighter, as if a weight has been lifted from their shoulders. Others recover more gradually, with an overall improvement that is punctuated by fewer and fewer bad days. Most feel well by three months, although a few residual symptoms, such as slowness in the mornings, may take longer to clear up.

People taking antidepressants usually want to stop them as soon as they feel better. But the risk of relapse is high for up to a year and most doctors recommend continuing the drugs for around four to six months after recovery. Then the antidepressants should be reduced gradually, not to avoid withdrawal symptoms, but because there is a risk of relapse as the drugs are cut down. For people with recurrent and severe depression, however, longer-term or even life-long treatment is safer. Those who would rather risk relapse should be offered regular support and ready access to help if things go wrong.

ELECTROCONVULSIVE THERAPY (ECT)

'What they do is' – McMurphy listens a moment – 'take some bird in there and shoot electricity through his skull?'

'That's a concise way of putting it.'

'What the hell for?'

'Why, the patient's good, of course . . . EST isn't always for punitive measures, as our nurse uses it, and it isn't pure sadism on the staff's part, either. A number of supposed Irrecoverables were brought back into

> contact with shock ... Shock treatment has some
> advantages; it's cheap, quick, entirely painless. It simply
> induces a seizure.'
> 'What a life,' Sefelt moans. 'Give some of us pills to
> stop a fit, give the rest shock to start one.'[12]

Electroconvulsive therapy (ECT), passing an electric current
through the brain to cause a fit or convulsion, is undoubtedly
the most controversial of the widely used psychiatric treatments. It seems crazy, unscientific, archaic, and even bar-
baric. Little is known about its effect on brain cells and brain
chemicals.

But ECT works, as has been borne out by many studies
comparing it favourably with antidepressants and placebo
treatments. More than four-fifths of severely depressed
people who have psychomotor retardation (mental slowing)
or delusions improve during a course of ECT. And, unlike
antidepressants, ECT starts to work immediately. Numerous
research studies show that at least two-thirds of people with
severe depression recover substantially within the first month
of ECT. This can be life-saving in people whose severe
depression is preventing them from eating and drinking or
is overwhelming them with suicidal feelings. Finally, the
treatment is safe – much safer than childbirth, for example.
The risk of dying during ECT is less than 0.1%, and the very
few deaths which do occur happen when the heart reacts
badly to the anaesthetic that is given with the treatment.

Despite these important benefits, ECT still has a bad name.
This is not simply a gut reaction against the nature of treatment, or against the lack of scientific understanding about
its actions. Its reputation has largely been tarnished by its
history.

Convulsions were first used to treat mental illness in the
1930s. The theory behind this was that people with epilepsy
never got schizophrenia and, therefore, inducing epileptic fits
would cure schizophrenia. The premise that epilepsy and
schizophrenia could not coexist was later shown to be untrue
but, in the absence of any effective drugs, ECT soon became

the mainstay of treatment for a wide range of mental health problems. In the initial years the treatment was given without anaesthetic to conscious patients. It caused unconsciousness immediately, then a full convulsion. As is the case in some epileptic fits, patients could thrash around and hurt themselves and even break bones. Strapping or holding them down often reduced the risk of injury, but it added to the apparent barbarism of the treatment. And before the Mental Health Act of 1959, ECT could be given to patients against their will without seeking a second opinion.

Things are very different now. Since the advent of antidepressant and antipsychotic drugs the use of ECT has narrowed and declined considerably. It is mostly reserved now for four conditions: depression that has not responded to antidepressants, life-threatening depression (i.e. with strong suicidal urges or with inability to eat and drink), depression in people whose physical health makes antidepressants too dangerous, and women with severe postnatal depression or psychosis. It is occasionally useful in unusual forms of schizophrenia and mania.

Treatment is usually given two or three times a week and, on average, eight times in all. Research on the best number of treatments or the ideal frequency per week is not conclusive; psychiatrists tend to prescribe courses according to severity and speed of recovery. Some people recover so quickly from their depression that they need only one or two treatments.

The treatment is given by two doctors. One, an anesthetist, injects into a vein (usually in the hand or arm) a short-acting anaesthetic drug and a muscle-relaxing drug that reduces the fit to twitching and minimizes the risk of injury to virtually zero. Oxygen is given by mask while the patient remains anaesthetized. The other doctor, a psychiatrist, places two electrodes on the patient's head. The electrodes deliver through the scalp about a tenth of the current used to restart the heart of someone who has had a cardiac arrest. The treatment takes about half a minute and the patient wakes from the anaesthetic within five or ten minutes.

Some people feel fine after treatment, others have a

ache or feel sick. Drowsiness, feeling muddled for a
hours, and an inability to remember what happened just
ore the treatment are all fairly common. Some, mostly
those who have responded quickly to ECT in the past and
have good support at home, come in as day patients for treatment. They are usually fit to go home a couple of hours later,
after tea and toast, as long as someone collects and looks after
them for the rest of the day.

Temporary confusion and memory loss are the main side
effects of ECT. People complain for up to a month that they
cannot clearly remember recent events and facts like phone
numbers and addresses. Very occasionally, some personal
memories are lost. Research on ECT's side effects is reassuring, showing that the vast majority of people suffer no permanent memory loss.

A survey published by the mental health charity MIND in
1993 showed that people who have had ECT tend to love it
or hate it.[13] Of the 516 people MIND surveyed, about half
had had ECT. Of these, 43% said it was 'helpful' or 'very
helpful' and 37% that it was 'unhelpful' or 'very unhelpful'.
Some condemned it strongly, saying that it was frightening.

Treatments for Specific Causes of Depression

TREATING POSTNATAL DEPRESSION AND OTHER
POSTNATAL MENTAL HEALTH PROBLEMS

Pregnant women who have had serious psychiatric illnesses
in the past should be offered preventive treatment around the
time of the baby's birth. They may need extra psychological
support at the outpatient clinic or at home, from a community
nurse or health visitor. They may also need drugs to keep
their mental state in balance and, if they are already on regular treatment, an increased dose may help. Most psychiatric
drugs are safe for the baby in pregnancy. But women should
check with their doctors to see that the drugs are safe as soon
as they discover that they are pregnant and must check again
if they decide to breastfeed.

The National Health Service routinely provides quite extensive support for mothers and their new babies. After the birth mothers are visited by specially trained community nurses for several weeks – first by midwives and later by health visitors. At about six weeks the GP examines the mother to see that she is recovering normally from childbirth. All of these checks provide chances for women to discuss any worries they have, and for the professionals to notice any signs of illness – both physical and psychological.

Most postnatal depression is fairly mild and is treatable by GPs. The organizations listed in Box 11 can also provide support and information. Women who need to see a psychiatrist will be treated as outpatients as far as possible, and every effort will be made not to disrupt family life and care of the baby. But if severe depression or psychosis develops, admission to hospital may be the safest option for the mother and the baby. In many parts of Britain the NHS offers special wards with nurses trained to care for both. Severe postnatal depression may need antidepressants and even ECT, which is often very effective.

Although psychiatric problems are triggered relatively easily by childbirth, those that are severe enough to need treatment are usually short-lived, clearing up within two or three months of onset. Postnatal psychotic illnesses usually resolve twice as quickly as those that are unrelated to pregnancy.

BOX 11

Sources of Help for Postnatal Depression
These organizations provide information and support:
National Childbirth Trust
Association of Post-Natal Illness
National Council for One Parent Families

TREATING DEPRESSION AT THE MENOPAUSE

For those women who become depressed at this time, usual antidepressant treatments – both psychological and physical – should help. There is no clear evidence that the hormonal changes of the menopause cause depression. But, because lack of female hormones – particularly oestrogen – is known to cause osteoporosis (bone thinning which predisposes to fractures) and circulatory and cardiac problems, many doctors now advocate postmenopausal hormone replacement therapy. Some women taking oestrogen find that it alleviates depression and increases feelings of wellbeing but, because the drug has widespread effects on the body, it is not usually recommended for psychological symptoms alone.

MANIC DEPRESSION

> The pending tray is empty when high, full when low; I want good weather so I can sail, ski, cycle, or play tennis when high. I welcome rain and bad weather forecasts when low. I welcome committee meetings when low: I destroy them when high. I love shopping when high: I cannot be bothered to buy my lunch when low. When high I catch the plane before the one I booked and flush the loo when only half finished . . . Overall there is the vicious paradox: I like myself when high but other people find it much easier to take me when I am low.[14]

Manic depression is usually a lifelong illness marked by recurrent episodes of severe depression and of abnormally elevated mood or mania. It affects just under 1% of the population in Britain, occurring more or less equally between the sexes. It usually starts at around 30. Alex's story is fairly typical:

> Alex, a 28-year-old factory worker, came under extra pressure at work to increase output. Although he was usually an efficient performer, worry about the increased demand made him start to lose concentration.

He took a couple of days off sick but things got worse. Over about three weeks Alex became irritable and, uncharacteristically, had several rows with his girlfriend at home.

Alex became preoccupied with weird and confused thoughts that the world was about to end. He heard voices in his head which he took to be God, giving him a mission to save mankind. Alex was convinced that he could do this because he had been filled with super-human skills of telepathy and power.

Life became increasingly disorganized. Alex felt too revved up to go to work, eat, or sleep: he was on the go day and night. He wrote copious notes on his new role, and went on long train journeys to check when the end of the world would come to different parts of the country.

One morning Alex had a sudden outburst of anger in the town centre. He had tried to buy every Ordnance Survey map for Great Britain and had threatened to hit the bookshop staff when they failed to provide them. The police were called. The officers realized immediately, on hearing Alex's confused defence of his behaviour and seeing how threatening he was, that he was ill and likely to harm himself or someone else.

The police took Alex to the police station, under the powers of the Mental Health Act, and called the GP whose turn it was to be police doctor. Alex told the doctor there was nothing wrong, indeed he felt on top of the world. Of course he couldn't go to hospital, said Alex, because he had to save the world.

By the end of that day Alex had been interviewed and examined by a psychiatrist and a social worker. His girlfriend came too and, despite wanting to help Alex herself, she said that she would feel threatened by him in his disturbed state. Reluctantly, but with some relief, she agreed that hospital would be the safest place for Alex. That evening Alex was admitted under the Mental Health Act to the local psychiatric unit.

Symptoms of Manic Depression

Confusingly, most psychiatrists call the highs hypomania, which simply means 'a bit less than completely manic'. They save the term mania for extremely elevated mood with severely disturbed and frenzied behaviour. Hypomanic people say they feel 'high, wonderful, better than they've ever felt before' and they can be warm, lovable, and fun to be with. But more often they are irritable, frustrated, and completely exhausting.

Hypomanic and depressive episodes last several months but during the gaps between them, which may last many years, sufferers are usually well. Many people with manic depression are able to continue with their careers and relationships, despite the strain of recurrent illness. Like depression, mania and hypomania can cause a mixture of psychological and physical symptoms (see Boxes 12 and 13).

BOX 12	**Psychological symptoms that may occur in mania and hypomania**
	Elated mood
	Manic thoughts
	extreme optimism
	inflated sense of self-importance
	unrealistic plans and schemes
	talking in puns and rhymes
	Psychotic symptoms
	hallucinations
	delusions

BOX 13

Physical symptoms that may occur in mania and hypomania
• Boundless energy
• Increased appetite
• Increased libido
• Insomnia
• Speeding up of actions and thoughts
• Poor concentration
• Distractibility
• Irritability
• Agitation
• Mental ⎫ particularly among confusion ⎭ elderly sufferers

Symptoms of Mania and Hypomania

Psychological Symptoms
Hypomanic people seem speeded up. Indeed, they may behave like people who have taken amphetamines or 'speed'. They think very quickly, but their minds are too revved up for ideas and conversation to form properly. They cannot concentrate and are easily distracted, flitting from thing to thing and going off at tangents. The apparent slowness of everyone else's thoughts and actions can irritate and anger hypomanic people, causing them to lose their temper easily.

Hypomanic people speak loudly, quickly, and profusely, making interruption difficult and often making others feel threatened. Sometimes, they speak in a curious linked, rhyming, or punning style which can seem very entertaining to casual observers. The content of hypomanic speech is typically grandiose, reflecting expansive thoughts and delusions.

Classically, hypomanic and manic people have delusions of grandeur. Alex, for instance, was convinced that he had special powers, had a vital mission for world peace, and was suddenly in touch with God. He also had grandiose hallucinations. Typically, he had no insight and neither acknowledged nor accepted the idea of being ill.

Hypomanic behaviour usually reflects the mood with restlessness, impatience, unpredictability, and inability to settle down to anything. Social inhibitions are flung away. Judgment and caution are impaired: sufferers might drive recklessly, make unwise decisions, and spend vast sums of money on unnecessary purchases or unrealistic schemes. Indeed, some hypomanic people jeopardize their whole family's finances.

Physical Symptoms

Hypomanic people are extremely restless. They can go for days on end without sleeping and can walk for miles on seemingly pointless journeys, wearing out their shoes. They may eat voraciously or, more commonly, be too busy and distracted to eat. Their libido may be increased.

Causes of Manic Depression

This illness is probably caused by many of the risk factors and precipitating factors that are thought to cause more straightforward depression (see Box 14). Heredity, however, seems to play a bigger part in causing manic depression.

BOX 14	**Probable causes of manic depression**
	Risk factors
	Inheritance
	Brain abnormalities
	Precipitating factors
	Psychological triggers

Life events

Physical triggers

Some physical illnesses

Childbirth

Steroids and amphetamines (can cause mania)

Risk Factors

Inheritance
More than two-thirds of identical twins of people with manic depression also develop the illness at some point in their lives. By contrast, about a fifth of non-identical twins will develop it. Thus the more genes a relative shares with a sufferer, the greater the risk of getting manic depression. Studies of manic depressive people who were adopted away from their natural families confirm that genes, rather than simply the childhood environment, are the main cause. Within sufferers' families some 10–15% of first-degree relatives – parents, children, and brothers and sisters – also develop the illness. Recent research suggests that the genetic abnormality probably lies in several chromosomes.

Some studies show that people with manic depression have an unusually high proportion of famous musicians, artists, performers, and writers in their families. And many famous people have actually had the illness. This suggests a hereditary link between manic depression and creativity – a credible theory, given the expansive and boundless thoughts experienced during hypomania.

Brain Abnormalities
Much less research has been done on possible brain abnormalities in manic depression than in schizophrenia. The little that has been done suggests that levels of the brain chemicals or neurotransmitters noradrenaline, serotonin, and dopam-

ine may all be altered. Some recent studies also show that certain parts of the brain use up glucose very quickly during hypomanic episodes. As is thought to be the case in schizophrenia and some types of depression, underlying genetic defects could cause these chemical abnormalities. On the other hand, a few experts think that stressful events and powerful emotions might trigger the chemical imbalances in otherwise normal brains.

Precipitating Factors

Both psychological and physical stresses can trigger first occurrences and relapses in manic depression. These include the factors already mentioned for depression plus some specific ones for hypomania and mania.

Psychological Triggers for Hypomania and Mania

LIFE EVENTS AND CHANGES

Several studies have shown that people admitted to hospital with episodes of hypomania and mania have experienced potentially stressful events in the preceding month. These are external events, not resulting from the illness. They are not all unpleasant and they range widely from moving house or organizing a wedding, to bereavement (see pp. 10–11 for a list of typical events).

MANIC THINKING

Aaron T. Beck, whose cognitive theory of depression is both popular and useful, says that over-optimistic and ego-boosting patterns of thinking can lead to mania and hypomania in susceptible people. As yet there is no widely used treatment based on this assumption, a cognitive therapy for mania.

Support for Beck's theory comes from observations that people who become hypomanic soon after episodes of depression somehow talk themselves into it. Certainly, some sufferers admit to staying up late, dieting, and misusing caffeine – by drinking huge amounts of coffee and cola – in risky attempts to get a little high and cheer themselves up.

PHYSICAL ILLNESS

Hypomania and mania can be triggered by many of the physical disorders that can cause depression, particularly childbirth. Some drugs, for example steroids and amphetamines, are known to dangerously elevate mood.

Treatment of Manic Depression

Treating Acute Attacks of Hypomania and Mania

The mainstays of treatment are a quiet, unstimulating environment and the same range of antipsychotic drugs that is used in schizophrenia (see Chapter 3). By and large, admission to hospital is the best way to provide the supervision and safety required, although mild hypomania can be treated in a day unit or at home if there is sufficient support.

Alex, who was described above, had to be taken to hospital against his will. He did not have to be manhandled there but on arrival he protested that he had to leave to get on with the important work God had given him. The ward doctor who interviewed and examined him explained that Alex could not leave. Although Alex did not appreciate that he was mentally ill, he agreed with the doctor's suggestion that a rest in hospital with some sedation, haloperidol, would help him to catch up on all the sleep he had missed recently.

The next day, once the first few doses of haloperidol had begun to work, Alex was more settled. Over the next week he did catch up on sleep, and on eating, and he became less preoccupied by his desire to leave hospital and continue his mission. At the end of four weeks in hospital the order detaining him there expired. By then Alex was beginning to accept that he had been very ill and he agreed to stay in hospital until he was well enough to go home.

The speed of recovery from hypomania is very variable, taking weeks or months. Sometimes the mood swings past the normal state and into depression. For some people this seems to be part of their inherent mood instability, but for others it seems to be an understandable response to the realization that they have been extremely ill with a problem that is likely to recur.

Most people recover fully from an attack of hypomania and are capable of picking up their lives where they left off. But some are reluctant to return to the stresses that may have caused the illness and decide to change their lifestyles accordingly. The degree of change needed is a personal choice, but it can be made with the support of family and friends and mental health staff.

Sufferers say that one of the hardest things about manic depression is fear of emotion. Lurking behind every happy time is the thought 'am I going too high?'

Long-Term Treatment for Manic Depression

A diagnosis of manic depression usually means that the sufferer will have intermittent attacks of hypomania or depression throughout life, interspersed by long periods of good health. Few sufferers need the intensive long-term care, such as special supervised accommodation, that those suffering from schizophrenia need. Many need reliable support and understanding, however, and so do their families and friends. The Manic Depression Fellowship is a national self-help organization and campaigning group. Its address is given in the directory in Appendix 2.

There is, however, no long-term cure for manic depression. But attacks can be made less frequent by continuing practical and psychological support and by long-term treatment with one of two drugs: lithium and carbamazepine.

LITHIUM

Lithium is the main preventive drug for manic depression and is occasionally given for persistent depression that does not respond to other treatments. Lithium is a naturally occurring element rather like sodium, the main constituent of salt. It is present in the body in tiny amounts with no known important biological function. Why lithium given as a drug stabilizes mood is not known either. Manic depression does not seem to be caused by lithium deficiency and lithium treatment is not a kind of replacement therapy. Nevertheless lithium does somehow control mood.

Several studies have shown that long-term lithium treatment greatly reduces the risk of relapse in around four-fifths of people with manic depression. For example, a study of nearly 250 long-term lithium users in New York found that 81% had good or fair mental health and that 56% had no episodes of mood disturbance over one year.[15] Before lithium and antipsychotic drugs were introduced, manic attacks lasted more than a year on average – and could last as long as ten years. The average now is about three months.

Some users of lithium say that it makes life seem rather grey and lacking in sparkle. It is hard to know if this is just their view of normal emotional experience, without the energy and enjoyment that a bit of hypomania can bring. Some, particularly those who rely strongly on their creativity, prefer to live with a relatively high risk of relapse than to take lithium.

A daily dose of lithium carbonate (trade names include Priadel and Camcolit) or lithium citrate (Litarex) is usually offered after two or more attacks of hypomania or after one each of hypomania and depression. Lithium may be suggested after only one episode of hypomania if the mood takes a long time to stabilize fully. Before starting lithium, patients must undergo a range of blood tests to ensure that they are fit to take it and that their kidneys and thyroid gland are working normally. This is because lithium can damage these organs, particularly if it becomes too concentrated in the blood. Therefore it should not be prescribed for people with kidney or thyroid problems.

Special care must be taken in prescribing lithium for people on other drugs. Dangerous interactions with lithium can occur with treatments for chest disease, heart disease, high blood pressure, and fluid retention. Specific drugs to avoid include water tablets (diuretics), steroids, and the antidepressants called SSRIs (p. 77). One drug that can be bought from chemists' counters without prescription, the pain killer ibuprofen (trade names Nurofen, Proflex, and Inoven), can be dangerous in large doses. Finally, high doses of the antipsychotic drug haloperidol should not be given to people on lithium because the combination seems to have caused a few cases of serious nerve and brain damage.

The risk that the level of lithium in the blood may become too high is minimized by simple measures (see Box 15). The most inconvenient and unpleasant of these measures is the need for regular blood tests. Urgent blood tests will be needed, too, if lithium's usually mild side effects (slight tremors, thirst, and increased urine flow) noticeably worsen or are added to by blurred vision, drowsiness, vomiting, and diarrhoea. These are early signs of lithium toxicity, when the concentration in the body rises to a dangerous level. At its worst, lithium toxicity can seriously affect the brain, nerves, kidneys and heart and can even kill. But clear instructions to users of lithium about the risks and signs of toxicity, regular tests, and stopping lithium immediately if warning signs appear all reduce the risk to almost nothing. Full-blown lithium toxicity is extremely rare, but all people offered lithium should have the risks fully explained so that they can weigh them up against the benefits.

BOX 15

Routine precautions to avoid lithium toxicity

- Take plenty of clear fluids, four or five pints of water a day and more in hot weather and after exercise

- Take tea, coffee, cola, and alcohol in moderation only

- Take a consistent amount of table salt – do not increase or reduce salt intake suddenly

- Have regular blood tests

- Always carry the treatment card that explains these precautions
- Stop lithium and seek medical advice immediately if you have diarrhoea or vomiting
- Stop lithium if any usual side effects worsen
- Finally, tell your doctor if you intend to become pregnant so that you can decide in advance whether to stop lithium

Lithium has one other danger: it can damage the unborn baby when taken in early pregnancy. If taken in late pregnancy lithium can also cause toxicity and thyroid disease in the newborn baby. Therefore, unless the likelihood of serious manic depressive relapse is so high that the mother's life is at risk, lithium should never be given in pregnancy. The best alternative is to remain drug free and allow frequent monitoring of mood by the GP, psychiatrist, or community nurse. If this is not possible, safe, low doses of carbamazepine (see below) or antipsychotic drugs can be given.

Lithium should be started as soon as the baby is born, however, because the risk of postnatal psychosis is high in women with manic depression. In theory, women taking lithium can breastfeed safely as long as the blood level is closely controlled. But in practice this may be difficult to do, given that breastfeeding mothers often fail to drink enough fluid. Therefore, women with manic depression who have just had babies should either forgo breastfeeding or lithium: a hard choice to make.

CARBAMAZEPINE
This drug, which is usually used to control epilepsy, can also stabilize mood. In manic depression carbamazepine is used mainly when lithium does not work well or when attacks occur very frequently, several times a year. It is less likely to be toxic than lithium, but its possible side effects include

blurred vision, unsteadiness, and dizziness at high doses. Although this drug has been used in epilepsy for many years now, it has been used in manic depression only in the past six or seven years, and not widely. There is, therefore, little research on its pros and cons in this illness.

3 SCHIZOPHRENIA

The Fragmented World

It was difficult to urge Philip on, to try to get over to him that eventually he would be well enough not to have to attend the hospital at all, and that it would all be worthwhile when that day arrived. Most of the time, however, it was not easy to reach Philip, for he was still only able to retain a little of what we said to him. Quite often he would seem almost to be in a trance-like state, staring into space, as though far, far away. And then there were the voices. It seemed as though they were never far away, but Philip denied that he could hear them when we asked if they were troubling him. With hindsight, I believe that in denying he could hear them, Philip was trying to put up a brave fight.

From *Schizophrenia: Voices in the Dark* by Mary Moate and David Enoch[1]

Schizophrenia is one of the most common and serious mental illnesses and one of the most misunderstood. Many people think, mistakenly, that a person with schizophrenia has a split personality, switching unpredictably like Dr Jekyll and Mr Hyde. In fact the word means split mind, and it is used to describe an illness in which the sufferer's inner world fragments. At its worst schizophrenia is an incurable, devastating example of what society sometimes calls madness and doctors call psychosis.

One reason why schizophrenia is difficult to understand is because it is not easy to define. It is a syndrome, or collection of symptoms and signs, that affects the mind and can alter thoughts, feelings, senses, motivations, and personality.

There is no test for schizophrenia: it is diagnosed when certain problems occur together and when the illness follows a certain course over time.

Some of the symptoms and signs of schizophrenia can also occur in other mental illnesses, for example in manic depression. Thus the diagnosis sometimes has to wait until the illness, its response to treatment, and its outcome can be observed, and other diseases have been ruled out. Psychiatrists often have to say to anxious relatives, 'We think it may be schizophrenia. We will treat the symptoms and do whatever else we can to help, and we will see what happens.' This may seem unsatisfactory, but it is an honest approach to diagnosis.

SCHIZOPHRENIA

Schizophrenia occurs in all countries and cultures around the world. Among people in developed countries the disorder occurs at roughly the same rate – about one in a hundred of the population get schizophrenia at some time during life. In developing countries schizophrenia tends to be slightly less common and less severe.

In the West schizophrenia usually starts in young adulthood (four-fifths of all sufferers become ill before they reach 45) and may appear suddenly, within a few days of a stressful event such as taking exams or starting college. More commonly, schizophrenia develops slowly over many months and the start is difficult to pinpoint. Stephen's story is typical:

> Stephen, a 19-year-old university student, unexpectedly did badly in his first term's exams. Little by little, he drifted out of friendships and the college's social life and spent increasing amounts of time alone in his room. He always seemed absorbed in thought but nothing much seemed to come of it: he was not obviously studying.
>
> Stephen told his curious and concerned friends that he was fine and wasn't worried about anything. But,

during his second term, he stopped attending lectures and became more and more withdrawn and strange. He was losing weight and, as far as anyone could see, he was no longer shaving or washing himself or changing his clothes. His tutor tried to find out what was wrong, but got nowhere: Stephen seemed almost afraid of her and wouldn't say much. But he agreed to see the college doctor.

The doctor sensed quickly that Stephen was mentally ill and asked some detailed direct questions about his experiences and symptoms. Stephen's replies were a bit difficult to follow because he seemed muddled and unable to concentrate. But he admitted yes, he was hearing voices when there was nobody there and, yes, he thought he was being controlled by some outside force. He firmly believed that some aliens had implanted an electronic device in his head while he was asleep, and that this enabled them to make him think and do certain things. This was, said Stephen, part of the aliens' plan to infiltrate society and take over the Earth. He knew that the aliens were getting very involved in national life because, reading between the lines, he could see that they were obviously responsible for many of the news stories reported in the press every day. He knew that they were preparing him for some as yet unspecified but special task because he had read messages to that effect in the number plates of his lecturers' cars. No, of course he wasn't imagining these ideas and sensations.

Further questions confirmed that Stephen firmly believed these strange ideas, or delusions. And it became clear that one of the reasons for his poor concentration was the almost continuous intrusion of the hallucinatory voices into his thoughts, even while the doctor was interviewing him. He admitted that this was making mundane things like eating and sleeping rather difficult, and that he was feeling very tired.

The doctor examined Stephen and found no signs of

physical illness. She was sure that Stephen was suffering from a serious mental illness, probably schizophrenia, and was worried that he would deteriorate quickly without treatment. To her relief, Stephen agreed to see a psychiatrist the following day, and subsequently took up the offer of a stay in hospital. Even though Stephen did not believe that he was ill, he admitted that he was tired and could do with a rest.

Schizophrenia often starts like this, gradually building up until it becomes so disturbing and debilitating that it cannot be missed or ignored. Work, relationships, and even basic things like eating and sleeping are interrupted so much that intensive practical help is needed every day. Such care can be, and often is, provided at home by relatives and friends. But, given that attacks of schizophrenia usually last many months and, given that regular doses of powerful drugs are usually needed to control the symptoms, doctors often recommend admission to psychiatric hospital.

Roughly a quarter of people who develop schizophrenia recover fully from their first attack without further consequences. They are said to have had acute (short-lived and transient) schizophrenia. Tragically, a quarter become disabled by chronic (long-term or permanent) schizophrenia and never recover or regain independent lives. The rest – one-half of all people who have an attack of schizophrenia – lie somewhere in between, often living independently but below the social and intellectual level expected from their earlier potential, and having lengthy relapses of acute illness every few years. Thus, sadly, for most sufferers schizophrenia is a long-term illness. This is one reason why people who have just one attack and recover fully may find that, as time goes on, doctors tell them it probably wasn't schizophrenia at all and was something much less serious. This can be very confusing and, not surprisingly, can make the whole process of diagnosis seem very unreliable. So, to make diagnosis as reliable as possible, doctors try to build up a detailed description of the sufferer's experiences, thoughts, and actions.

Signs and Symptoms of Schizophrenia

The Acute Illness

The experiences at the height of an attack of schizophrenia usually dominate the sufferer's whole world. They may be very strange, almost incomprehensible to anyone else. One way of trying to understand these experiences and the way they interlink is to group them together (see Box 1). Psychiatrists separate them into disturbances of perception, thought, emotion, and awareness of reality. The ability to judge what is real is also damaged. And all of these disturbances can alter behaviour, making sufferers seem strange and obviously unwell.

BOX 1

Symptoms of Schizophrenia
The following may be disturbed:
Perception – with hallucinations (mainly voices)
Thought – with thought disorder and delusions
Emotion – often flattened
Self-awareness – with feelings of being invaded or controlled
Reality awareness – with inability to discern what is real and no insight into being ill
Behaviour – with poor self-care, agitation or lethargy; committing strange acts, but rarely with violence

DISTURBANCES OF PERCEPTION

All of the senses can be affected by hallucinations, which are perceptions that seem absolutely real but have no external cause. The commonest type in schizophrenia affect hearing and are called auditory hallucinations.

Sufferers usually say that they hear voices or noises that come from inside or outside their heads but have no visible source. The voices may be single or multiple, speaking directly to the sufferer or to each other. They may mutter unintelligibly. Sometimes, and often more disturbingly, the voices make very clear statements and comments that insult, direct, or describe the sufferer and his or her actions and thoughts. These experiences can threaten the normal sense of a personal boundary where the self ends and others begin, and are often accompanied by delusions that everyone else can read or control the sufferer's mind.

Auditory hallucinations can be very distracting and can interrupt tasks and conversations. Some sufferers believe that the voices are coming from real people around them, and try to respond to them. We have all seen obviously disturbed people who shout at strangers in the street: most do this because they hear hallucinatory voices.

Although auditory hallucinations are by far the commonest type in schizophrenia, other senses may also be affected. And, like auditory hallucinations, other kinds of hallucination can tie in with delusions. Strange smells and tastes often occur with delusions about being poisoned, weird bodily sensations often accompany delusions of being physically controlled like a puppet or robot. Visual hallucinations (of which some religious visions are thought to be examples) are less common.

Because they are not real, hallucinations do not always follow the normal rules of perception: a voice may be located in the chest, and objects may be seen to move in and out of the body through intact skin ('The voices started in my mouth and moved to six inches in front of my face. It's my mother and father. Sometimes they're friendly, sometimes they shout.'). Thus hallucinations are sometimes said to have a dreamlike quality. Nightmarelike might be a better term.

DISTURBANCES OF THOUGHT
Schizophrenia affects the way thoughts are processed, preventing sufferers from thinking straight. The problem, called thought disorder, is usually detectable in speech. Conver-

sation does not hang together and veers off the point or suddenly stops. Mild thought disorder can be difficult to spot, and listeners may think that their own concentration is poor. More severe disorder can produce strange, lyrical speech and made-up words (called neologisms) that only just make sense. Dylan Thomas used a similar style in his play *Under Milk Wood*:

> Lord Cut-Glass, in his kitchen full of time, squats down alone to a dogdish, marked Fido, of peppery fish-scraps and listens to the voices of his sixty-six clocks that cataract their ticks, old time-weeping with love, their black-and-white moony loudlipped faces tocking the earth away . . .[2]

As well as affecting the processing of thought, schizophrenia can alter its content, producing false beliefs called delusions. Delusions are more than just funny ideas or the products of a fertile imagination. They are firm, often complicated, beliefs that go against common sense and remain firm even when challenged by evidence that shows them to be untrue. In fact, hard evidence isn't usually necessary to convince other people that someone is deluded because delusional ideas are usually so incongruous and out of keeping with the sufferer's past and present life that they are patently untrue. For example, an English-born farmer with schizophrenia might develop delusions about the CIA following him and tapping his phone, even though he had never been to the USA and had never done anything that might warrant such attention. These surprising and highly unlikely beliefs would be unshakeable, even if his friends and family had much more logical and mundane explanations for every incident that made him think he was being followed and even if there was no evidence that his phone was being tapped.

Delusions may come out of the blue, suddenly imparting new knowledge. They may also fit closely with and, perhaps, follow on from hallucinations: for instance, someone with delusions of persecution might have heard voices discussing ways of harming him. Delusions may also develop from misinterpretations of ordinary events; cars passing by the sufferer's house at night might be misconstrued as evidence of being spied on, and news stories in the media might be taken as unusually and personally meaningful. 'I don't watch the TV because the people keep telling me I am sinful. I often write to the BBC about it – they've known about me for years'. Stephen, who is described above, had delusions about being controlled by aliens and had the related idea that the television and newspapers were confirming his experiences. And he had attached false significance to something very ordinary; a few car number plates.

DISTURBANCES OF EMOTION
The experiences that occur in schizophrenia may, understandably, make sufferers feel intensely fearful, perplexed, suspicious, angry, or depressed. But they often seem to have quite inappropriate emotions, being unperturbed or even cheerful when describing symptoms that most people would find distressing. Some people with schizophrenia seem to develop flattened or blunted emotions, which makes them unable to experience the normal range of human feelings. This may just mean that a certain edge or sparkle goes from the personality, but it can lead to a void of apathy, particularly when the illness lasts a long time: Jean, 61, was very difficult to motivate to do anything except sit in her chair. She was reluctant to bathe or change her clothes and seemed to have lost the capacity for active involvement and enjoyment in things.

DISTURBANCES OF SELF-AWARENESS
Healthy people usually have a clear sense of self, knowing the difference between the inner world of their own thoughts and feelings and the outside world of other people and things. Among people with schizophrenia this sense of self often breaks down.

Sufferers sometimes feel that their actions are no longer their own but are actively controlled by some outside person or force. This feeling of passivity can affect simple physical actions, such as blinking or walking, making the sufferer feel like a puppet. It can also extend to much more complicated actions, motivations, and thought processes. Some sufferers believe they have developed a kind of telepathy, so that their thoughts are accessible to or are inserted into their minds by others.

DISTURBANCE OF REALITY AWARENESS

It is fairly common for healthy people to experience things that are not real. For instance, someone taking a short cut home through a cemetery at night might think that a bush up ahead is a person waiting in the shadows. But reality will intervene and show the bush to be just a bush as the walker approaches it. And a conscientious and hard-working exam candidate with little self-confidence may be convinced of failure, until the letter arrives to say he or she has passed. In schizophrenia, as in other psychoses, the ability to tell what is real is impaired. The hallucinations, delusions, and other disturbances all seem completely real, even when other people try to explain them as symptoms of illness. Sufferers are so convinced of the reality of their experiences that they often do not accept that they are ill: Maurice, 51, firmly believed that intruders were getting into his flat and stealing minor household objects, even though there was no sign of forced entry and he had changed the locks four times.

DISTURBANCES OF BEHAVIOUR

All the disturbances that occur in schizophrenia can affect behaviour. Sufferers often try to follow what their senses and thoughts tell them, acting on their hallucinations and delusions. For example, Stephen, who was described above, bought every daily newspaper for many weeks so that he could closely follow the aliens' activities. His room was stuffed with piles of old newspapers.

Schizophrenia's more general effects on behaviour include altered energy level (lethargy or, less often, agitation), poor social skills (becoming withdrawn and shy or socially odd), and poor self-care (loss of interest in personal hygiene,

appearance, shopping, and cooking). For these reasons sufferers often need a great deal of practical help in living their
lives.

Occasionally, acute attacks of schizophrenia can make
people aggressive and violent. This may be self-directed, end-
ing in self-injury or suicide. Very occasionally the aggression
is directed at others. Although such tragedies attract understandable concern, the resulting publicity is usually misleading and cruelly stigmatizing, suggesting that schizophrenia
commonly makes people dangerous. In fact, quite the opposite is true, given that schizophrenia usually causes apathy
and lethargy. More than 200,000 people in Britain have
schizophrenia, yet only a handful of press reports each year
document violent behaviour by sufferers.

The Chronic Illness

The severe disturbance and alarming symptoms of acute
schizophrenia usually wane with time and treatment. Sufferers who go on to develop chronic schizophrenia may be
left with shadowy versions of their acute symptoms – they
may hear the odd voice or express strange ideas at times. But
they are also left with shadowy versions of themselves, and
this is the most disabling aspect of the chronic illness. Something strikes at the personality, causing apathy and a kind of
emptiness of thought and emotion. Warmth, humour, spon-
taneity, and some essential part of individuality are lost. Tom,
47, completed two years at university before becoming ill;
now his life revolves around his next cigarette, his belief that
he is king of a foreign country, and performance of his daily
chores in the hostel where he lives.

Psychiatrists sometimes describe the symptoms of chronic
schizophrenia as 'negative', reflecting the overwhelming
impression that it is a state of loss. By contrast, the florid
symptoms of the acute illness are described as 'positive'.
These are not value judgments and do not equate with bad
and good; they just reflect the active or passive nature of
certain symptoms.

Causes of Schizophrenia

It is, perhaps, one of the greatest failures of modern science that the cause of schizophrenia is still unknown. Most doctors and scientists believe that two groups of factors explain how schizophrenia arises: firstly, there are risk factors that cause the tendency to develop the illness and, secondly, there are precipitating factors that trigger attacks.

Thus far, scientific research has come up with two main risk factors – heredity and brain abnormality – and one main precipitating factor – stress – which has several causes in turn (see Box 2).

BOX 2

Possible causes of schizophrenia
Risk factors
inheritance
brain abnormalities
Precipitating factors
stress
recreational drugs

Risk Factors

INHERITANCE

Schizophrenia sometimes runs in families – about one in five sufferers has at least one relative who also has the illness. Those relatives whose genetic make-up is closest to that of the sufferer are more likely to develop schizophrenia themselves in future than are more distant relatives. Research on many families has shown a consistent pattern, making it possible to estimate approximate risks for relatives (see Box 3). Thus the child of a parent with schizophrenia has about a one in eight chance of developing the illness at some time in the future. If both parents have schizophrenia, the risk for each child is one in two.

BOX 3

Approximate risks of developing schizophrenia for different relatives of a sufferer	
	%
Identical twin	50
Child of two affected parents	50
Non-identical twin	17
Child of one affected parent	12
Non-twin brother or sister	8
Half brother or sister	3
Nephew or niece	2

The fact that schizophrenia runs in some families suggests that the illness may be at least partly due to a problem in the natural genetic processes of inheritance. But identical twins of sufferers, who have exactly the same genes as their twins, do not always develop the disease; thus inheritance cannot be the whole answer. Perhaps something in the physical and emotional environment during childhood is important in affected families. One way to sort out the differing effects of nature and nurture in schizophrenia is to study relatives who have become separated from sufferers in childhood and have thereby had different upbringings in different places.

Several researchers have looked at adopted children whose biological parents had schizophrenia but whose adoptive parents did not. These children developed schizophrenia more often than other adopted children. By the same token, children whose adoptive parents later develop schizophrenia but whose biological parents do not are at no greater risk than their peers. Both kinds of research support the theory that genetic inheritance, rather than upbringing, increases the risk of getting schizophrenia.

Inheritance might explain one other pattern in the incidence of schizophrenia. A huge body of research has shown that schizophrenia is much more commonly diagnosed among Afro-Caribbean people in Britain than in white people or any other ethnic group. Maybe schizophrenia is inherited along with ethnicity, in similar ways to blood disorders like sickle cell disease and thalassaemia.

One recent study in Manchester found that the rate for schizophrenia among black people born in Britain was nine times higher than among white people.[3] The authors discussed one of the main criticisms of this recurrent finding: namely that it is a result of misdiagnosis, based on Eurocentric and ultimately racist ideas about black culture and behaviour. This may well be the case, given that Afro-Caribbean patients are much more likely than other groups to be admitted by the police under the Mental Health Act. In turn, however, the Manchester study suggested that black people are less likely than white or Asian people to seek medical help and are more likely to become very disturbed before reaching the psychiatric services. Another explanation is that the schizophrenia-like symptoms are transient and do not warrant hospital care or drug treatment because they are caused by cannabis, which many Afro-Caribbeans use regularly. Finally, the stresses of migration, a different culture, and racial discrimination may be more than enough to precipitate schizophrenia in Afro-Caribbean people in Britain. The Manchester study did not support this idea, however, because the Asian people studied had suffered similar stresses without developing schizophrenia at the same high rate.

Thus, the reasons behind so-called 'black schizophrenia' are not known. As yet, there is no genetic evidence to explain it. But, at the moment, there is only the most basic of genetic explanations for anyone getting schizophrenia. Beyond saying that the risk of getting schizophrenia is at least partly transmitted by inheritance, little else is known conclusively about which of the building blocks or genes that make up chromosomes might be faulty or about what is passed on (perhaps a chemical or anatomical abnormality in the brain). One favoured theory is that the vulnerability for schizophrenia is carried in several faulty genes and people with most or all of these genes are particularly likely to succumb to the illness in certain circumstances. Many researchers think that great progress will be made in the next few years, as a result of work done by the international Human Genome Project. The project is a detailed and highly technical study of the whole range of human genes which has already found the cause of several hereditary diseases such as Huntington's disease (see p. 149) and certain types of muscular dystrophy.

Up till now, detecting that someone has a faulty gene before they develop the related physical abnormality has had two main uses. Firstly, detection among children and adults means they can be counselled and better prepared for their future problems. Secondly, detection of serious genetic disorders among unborn babies means that parents can choose to terminate the pregnancies. In future, however, early detection will allow prevention and treatment of genetic disorders by gene therapy. This has already been done: in 1991 a four-year-old girl with a fatal genetic disorder had healthy genes inserted into cells of her body, which replaced her faulty genes and corrected her disease. There is a small possibility that gene therapy could prevent schizophrenia in future.

BRAIN INJURIES AND ABNORMALITIES
Special brain scans (see p. xxii) show that some people with chronic schizophrenia have both anatomical and chemical abnormalities in the temporal lobes of the brain (the brain regions that handle and interpret information coming in from outside via the senses). Specialists in brain development and function believe that these abnormalities occur in very early life but do not cause the problems of schizophrenia until the brain rapidly matures in young adulthood. These acquired brain abnormalities could explain the four-fifths of sufferers who develop the illness out of the blue, without any record of schizophrenia running in their families.

These abnormalities could be inherited. But there is some evidence that they are acquired during pregnancy or around the time of birth. For example, a study of Irish maternity records found that babies who developed schizophrenia in adulthood were much more likely than other babies to have had birth complications needing obstetric intervention.[4] This did not mean, however, that the interventions such as forceps delivery caused the schizophrenia. The babies needed extra help because they had fetal distress (lack of oxygen to the heart and brain) during otherwise normal labours. This suggested that they already had abnormalities that made them particularly vulnerable to the trauma of being born.

One other main cause for these brain abnormalities has been suggested by research: viral infection and antenatal or birth complications. One study in England and Wales found that young adults getting schizophrenia in the 1970s would have been fetuses of three to seven months (that is, their mothers would have been in the middle stages of pregnancy) when big national epidemics of influenza occurred.[5] The implication is that the mothers had flu and passed it on to their developing babies, damaging their growing brains. But whether those mothers actually caught flu was not recorded, and another similar study found no link between mothers' flu and offsprings' schizophrenia. The second study documented actual cases of flu among mothers of 17,000 babies born in Britain in a single week in 1958. Follow up of those babies found that they were no more at risk of schizophrenia in adulthood than those whose mothers did not get flu in pregnancy. No link was found with birth complications, either.[6]

While research on the causes of these brain abnormalities continues, other scientists are looking at the way in which the abnormalities might in turn cause schizophrenia. One possibility is that they cause faulty 'wiring' in the brain, so that the wrong electrical impulses are sent to the wrong places and the brain malfunctions. Some support for this idea comes from studies showing that epilepsy, a brain disorder known to be caused by faulty wiring, is sometimes associated with schizophrenia. Another related idea is that the abnormalities disrupt the next component of the brain's communications network; the chemical messengers or neurotransmitters. These chemicals, released by the action of nerve impulses, do the real work of the brain – making perceptions, thoughts, and actions happen. When their production and balance is disrupted the brain malfunctions. In schizophrenia certain brain chemicals, including dopamine and serotonin, are known to be affected.

Precipitating Factors

Like the research on the early risk factors that might make people vulnerable to schizophrenia, studies on the immediate precipitants of first attacks have proved surprisingly difficult. But the large body of conflicting research done so far has come up with one broad theory: many people first develop schizophrenia after a particularly important life event, such as emigrating, having a baby, or starting college. (Stephen, the student described on pp. 98–100, had recently started college when he became ill.)

The assumption is that psychological and social stress tends to precipitate schizophrenia among adults who are already predisposed to the illness. But the link between stress and the first attack is not always clear.

For a small proportion of sufferers one factor – recreational drug use – seems much more definitely linked to onset of schizophrenia. Amphetamines and hallucinogens, which can cause transient hallucinations and delusions in any user, are particularly dangerous for people who are prone to schizophrenia. Cannabis is also thought to trigger schizophrenia in some cases.

Factors Which Do Not Cause Schizophrenia

Thirty or forty years ago research on schizophrenia was concentrated on trying to find a purely social cause, particularly within sufferers' families. Terms like the 'schizophrenogenic mother' were widely used to blame mothers for making their children ill. And schizophrenia was said to result solely from confusion caused by a family atmosphere of contradictory messages or 'double binds'; for instance, a child given very little affection or attention by his parents might be told, perfunctorily and unconvincingly, that they loved him.

The work of one Scottish psychiatrist and psychoanalyst, R. D. Laing, was widely endorsed during the 1960s and 70s. Laing did not accept that schizophrenia was a mysterious brain illness; he argued that it was a logical response to a sick family and emotionally unhealthy upbringing. In *Sanity*,

Madness and the Family Laing and his fellow psychiatrist Aaron Esterson said:

> When a psychiatrist diagnoses schizophrenia, he means that the patient's experience and behaviour are disturbed because there is something the matter with the patient that causes the disturbed behaviour he observes. He calls this something schizophrenia, and he then must ask what causes the schizophrenia . . .
>
> Though the term has now been generally adopted and psychiatrists trained in its application, the fact that it is supposed to denote remains elusive. Even two psychiatrists from the same medical school cannot agree on who is schizophrenic independently of each other more than eight out of ten times at best . . .
>
> We set out to illustrate that, if we look at some experience and behaviour without reference to family interactions, they may appear comparatively socially senseless, but that if we look at the same experience and behaviour in their original family context they are liable to make more sense.[7]

More recent research has discredited these earlier theories: people with schizophrenia do not have stranger or more disrupted families than anyone else. Yet relatives, particularly parents, often blame themselves when young people become mentally ill, and many are still made to feel guilty by the remnants of the old theories.

Despite increasing evidence that serious mental illnesses are caused by brain disease, the critics of mainstream psychiatry still command wide audiences. Like Laing, Thomas S. Szasz, a Hungarian who became a psychiatrist in the USA in 1946, also challenged the idea that schizophrenia is a brain illness and argued that the medical concept of mental illness is wrong. Szasz, however, blamed society rather than the family for the problem. He said that society, and psychiatrists in particular, use the term mental illness as a stigmatizing label for people whose behaviour annoys or offends others. Analogies to bodily illness and to treatments and cures were spurious, he said, because they hid the real personal and social problems of 'sick' people and absolved them of responsibility for their actions. In his book *The Myth of Mental Illness* Szasz argued:

> I submit that the traditional definition of psychiatry, which is still in vogue, places it alongside such things as alchemy and astrology, and commits it to the category of pseudo-science.[8]

For some of the less serious conditions that psychiatrists include under the wide definition of mental illness, both Laing and Szasz may have good points. And, even in schizophrenia, research has shown repeatedly that emotional factors in families can trigger relapses in people with the chronic illness (pp. 129–31). But it is very hard to believe that the underlying problem in schizophrenia and the gravely disrupting nature of a first attack can have any cause other than a physical brain disease. Widespread social and medical research has not borne out Laing's and Szasz's theories.

Treatment of Schizophrenia

BOX 4

Treating schizophrenia

Treatment for acute attacks:
- Support and supervision in unstimulating environment
- Antipsychotic drugs, by mouth or injection
- Drugs to counteract side effects
- Occupational therapy
- Rehabilitation

After discharge:
- Care programmes run by care managers and key workers
- Avoiding family stress

- Antipsychotic drugs by depot injections or tablets
- Drugs to counteract side effects

The overwhelming nature of an acute schizophrenic illness means that medical treatment, both with drugs and intensive practical support, is nearly always needed (see Box 4). Stephen, the student whose schizophrenic breakdown was described earlier in this chapter, stayed in hospital for seven months.

Stephen was admitted to a large psychiatric hospital near his college. It was a huge old building with long corridors and draughty wards and his ward was full of strange people. But Stephen felt safer there than he had done at college and he found that both patients and staff seemed to understand what he'd been going through.

The ward doctor, who had seen Stephen on admission and had asked him a seemingly endless list of questions, prescribed some tablets to take every morning and night. Although Stephen didn't think he was ill, he felt tired and a bit odd. So he took the tablets, and he continued to take them even though they made his mouth dry and his hands shake. He slept better and began to feel hungrier than he had done for weeks.

Stephen's parents came to visit him. They seemed very worried and a bit paranoid, he thought. But it was nice of them to come. They brought him some books and magazines, but he didn't feel like reading. At first Stephen spent most of his time sitting in the day room. Sometimes he stared at the television, sometimes he talked to other people. But he spent much of the time just sitting and not doing much. He still felt that he was being controlled by aliens, although it was harder for them to get to him now that there were people around all the time. He still heard the voices.

After a week Stephen felt much more interested in what was going on around him. He wanted to watch television but the picture was blurred, and he felt too sleepy to read. He started getting to know some of the other people on the ward, particularly one guy who was only a year older than him who had also dropped out of college. He also talked to the nurses more, and told them how tired he was feeling. The next day Stephen's medication was reduced and he soon felt much less sleepy.

Over the next five months Stephen gradually recovered. His symptoms lessened and his concentration improved little by little. He no longer had to take tablets regularly because he had a monthly injection that gave the same amount of medication more slowly, although he had episodes of hand-trembling every few days and had to take a few tablets then.

He attended occupational therapy, building up to going four days a week, working on the word processor and cooking regularly. When his friends from college visited he went out to the local shops and pubs with them, although he was on strict instructions not to drink more than a pint. Stephen began to talk about going back to college.

The first step, however, was to try going home. At first Stephen wasn't keen on the idea because he wanted to go back to college straight away and his parents lived about 80 miles away. But he could still barely concentrate to read a whole newspaper and he still talked sometimes about the aliens and their continued interference in his life. And the college said that Stephen was welcome to come back at the beginning of the next academic year, 11 months away. He accepted the offer, and agreed to spend the next year at home.

After several successful days and weekends at home Stephen was discharged. His care was transferred to a mental health team in his home town and he was offered a regular place at a day centre where he could practise writing essays on the word processor. He continued his medication over the next year, and his delusions disappeared completely. He still heard voices at times, particularly when he was not doing much. But they no longer bothered him. Sadly, Stephen's abilities to concentrate and learn did not return to their previous levels and he did not go back to college. Instead he started work as a clerical assistant in a local office, and a year later he left home to live with some friends.

Stephen took many months to recover from his schizophrenic attack with a mixture of medical and practical help. He was not cured completely and he continued with drug treatment, but he was able to pick up his life on leaving hospital.

Drug Treatment

As yet, there is no cure for schizophrenia, and current treatments can cause unpleasant side effects. But the mainstay of treatment, a group of drugs used since the early 1950s, has done much to alleviate the symptoms and allow many patients to leave psychiatric hospitals and take up more independent lives outside. The group of drugs is known by three names – antipsychotics, major tranquillizers, or neuroleptics.

Despite being called major tranquillizers, only some of these drugs have a tranquillizing effect on people with schizophrenia. This sedation can help in acute attacks, calming the frightened or agitated sufferer and encouraging much-needed sleep. Thus the most sedative drugs in the group, such as chlorpromazine, are often used at the start of treatment and in emergencies. Other drugs in the group that are much less sedative include trifluoperazine, pimozide, and haloperidol. They are particularly used for people whose illnesses have made them lethargic and apathetic.

More importantly, the antipsychotics damp down the symptoms of schizophrenia; particularly the hallucinations and delusions. They are thought to do this by blocking the activity of dopamine, the chemical messenger in the brain that seems to go wrong in schizophrenia. Antipsychotic drugs also hasten and prolong remission (the term doctors use for the gap between attacks in any relapsing illness). Thus, sufferers from chronic schizophrenia are usually advised strongly to take the drugs indefinitely.

For short-term treatment of acute schizophrenia drugs are usually given by tablet or liquid form, with fast-acting injections in emergencies. Tablets have to be taken several times a day, a daunting prospect if treatment is eventually needed for months or even years. But there is an alternative for people who need long-term treatment – long acting 'depot' injections, usually given by a nurse at three to four week intervals. This saves the sufferer from having to remember to take tablets and it ensures regular, medically monitored, treatment. Depot injections do not usually hurt, and complications such as inflammation and nodules at the site of injection (mainly the buttock) are rare.

SIDE EFFECTS OF ANTIPSYCHOTIC DRUGS
Sadly, like most potent drugs, antipsychotics can have unwanted and sometimes disabling side effects (see Box 5). Some of these, such as dizziness on standing up, blurred vision, dry mouth, constipation, and weight gain, can be avoided by keeping the dose as low as possible.

Other side effects – shaking, stiff posture, and limb restlessness like those occurring in Parkinson's Disease – may be harder to control by adjusting the dose. But they can be counteracted by taking a different type of drug such as procyclidine (brand name Kemadrin) or benzhexol (Artane). And all of these side effects can often be avoided by trying different members of the antipsychotic drug family (see Box 6).

BOX 5

Side Effects of Antipsychotic Drugs

Common avoidable or treatable effects include:

- Dizziness
- Blurred vision
- Dry mouth
- Constipation
- Weight gain
- Shaking
- Stiffness
- Limb restlessness
- Discolouration of skin when exposed to the sun

In the long term about a fifth of people on antipsychotic drugs get some degree of tardive dyskinesia:

Abnormal movements of face, trunk, and limbs

Abnormal walking

BOX 6

Examples of antipsychotic drugs*

Drugs given by mouth or short-acting injection
Those that cause sedation

- Chlorpromazine (Largactil), high dose sulpiride (Dolmatil)

Those that cause only moderate sedation

- Thioridazine (Melleril), pimozide (Orap), perphenazine (Fentazin)

* Brand names given in brackets

Those that cause little sedation

- Trifluoperazine (Stelazine), haloperidol (Haldol, Serenace), low-dose sulpiride (Dolmatil)

Drugs given by long-acting depot injection

- Flupenthixol decanoate (Depixol)

- Fluphenazine decanoate (Modecate)

- Zuclopenthixol decanoate (Clopixol)

- Haloperidol decanoate (Haldol Decanoate)

During acute attacks of schizophrenia, when the drugs are having considerable benefit, side effects often seem relatively unimportant. But some sufferers, their relatives, and even their doctors, find these unwanted effects much less bearable during periods of remission, even when medication has been reduced. One solution is to stop the medication under close medical supervision. These 'drug holidays', however, are risky because they increase the chance of relapse (see pp. 128–9). Thus, doctors tend to recommend such treatment breaks only to people who agree to close supervision and whose relapses are easy to foresee and stall.

Doctors should take particular care in prescribing antipsychotic drugs for elderly people, for whom both the risk and severity of side effects can be dangerous. Dizziness and unsteadiness, often mild and transient side effects in younger people, may make fragile old people fall and hurt themselves badly. And disturbed body temperature regulation, which can cause extremely rare but potentially serious overheating (malignant hyperthermia) in younger people on antipsychotics, can cause both hypothermia and hyperthermia in older people. Finally, the risk of antipsychotic-induced shaking and stiffness is higher in old age, when Parkinson's Disease is commonest anyway. Among elderly people, who often get quite mild psychotic symptoms, the drugs' side effects can outweigh their benefits. Thus, although these side effects can be reversed, they should not be allowed to occur in the first place unless the schizophrenia is very severe.

Tardive dyskinesia So much for reversible side effects that occur during treatment. A more worrying, sometimes irreversible, type of side effect called tardive dyskinesia occurs in about a fifth of people taking long-term medication with antipsychotics. And it can occur months or even years after treatment has stopped.

Tardive dyskinesia describes a syndrome or group of abnormal movements affecting the face (grimacing, for example), trunk, and limbs (odd walking patterns and postures). Sufferers have very limited control over the movements, and are not always aware of them. In many people tardive dyskinesia is, thankfully, mild and barely noticeable. And in many it stops completely when the antipsychotics are reduced or stopped.

But for some people tardive dyskinesia is disfiguring and disabling. Thus, avoiding it is a high priority in psychiatric treatment. Because elderly people and those who have taken antipsychotics for many years are most likely to get it, doctors should avoid continuous prescriptions for older people with schizophrenia or make sure that they are monitored very closely by a psychiatrist, a GP, or a psychiatric nurse.

There is one other way to avoid tardive dyskinesia when treating schizophrenia – by using clozapine. Clozapine is an antipsychotic that was first used over 30 years ago and in more than 30 countries worldwide. Uniquely among effective anti-schizophrenia drugs, clozapine does not cause tardive dyskinesia. But up to half of all people who take it suffer side effects that can include sedation, overproduction of saliva, weight gain, heart abnormalities, and even seizures. Much more drastically, clozapine killed 16 patients in the 1970s by blocking the production of white blood cells in their bone marrow. Because of this, clozapine was taken off the market in many countries, including Britain.

Since 1989 clozapine has been available again in Britain, but only for patients with severe schizophrenia that has not responded to anything else, and only with regular blood tests to pick up any fall in the white cell count at an easily treatable stage. Patients on clozapine (which is available only by mouth, not as a long-acting depot injection) now have to have blood tests every week for the first 18 weeks of treatment and fortnightly after that. This treatment and testing regime is expensive, costing an average £2000 a year per patient at 1993 prices, compared with about £60 a year for a monthly depot injection of another major tranquillizer. But studies of overall costs suggest that clozapine is good value because patients taking it need much less psychiatric help in the long run. The next step is to find a safe drug that works as well as clozapine.

Psychological and Practical Aspects of Treatment

IN HOSPITAL

People suffering acute attacks of schizophrenia are usually too disturbed and muddled to cope with any kind of talking therapy or occupational therapy. Their main need is for a safe, quiet, and relatively unstimulating environment staffed by carers who are reassuring, informative, willing to listen, and helpful. These are the ingredients of a good psychiatric ward or day hospital, but can also be provided at home or in sheltered accommodation if enough experienced carers are available.

In hospital psychiatric nurses provide the bulk of such care. Nurses listen and talk to patients individually, and help them to focus on daily realities like self-care and current affairs rather than psychotic preoccupations. Nurses can help patients regain their concentration by, for example, playing board games. Muddled thinking, disturbed behaviour, and social withdrawal can be lessened by participation in communal meetings and in ward routines such as preparing the dining room for meals. Most nurses would wish to work to these standards, but individual care is difficult to maintain when staffing levels are so low that a couple of nurses have to cater for up to 30 patients.

Individual care can change gear once recovery gets under-way and the psychotic symptoms begin to fade. As the hal-lucinations quieten and the sense of self becomes more solid, the demands of the world outside hospital can be reintro-duced gradually. The recovering patient can start occupa-tional therapy and begin to make plans with friends, family, or a social worker for accommodation and, perhaps, employment.

A well-run occupational therapy department should offer individually tailored programmes of regular constructive activities. These activities should allow the therapists to assess patients' needs and encourage patients to regain the concentration, confidence, and independence that are often shattered by psychotic illnesses. Suitable activities include domestic independence skills (cooking, budgeting, shop-ping), work retraining (such as keyboard skills), literacy edu-cation, creative arts, horticulture, group therapy, and training to cope with anxiety.

PREPARING FOR DISCHARGE FROM HOSPITAL
Schizophrenic attacks usually last many weeks and months. Acute positive symptoms such as hallucinations and delusions usually start to recede after a week or two on medi-cation. Patients often notice that the hallucinatory voices get fainter and less frequent, and they become gradually less preoccupied by and less convinced about their delusional ideas.

When and if the symptoms of acute schizophrenia com-pletely stop many patients recall them only hazily. Some who regain insight, understanding that the experiences were part of an illness rather than external reality, feel too embarrassed and distressed to talk about them. This distress, and the realization that schizophrenia usually recurs throughout life, can lead, understandably, to depression. Other sufferers continue to believe that the experiences were real and simply say that the external interference in their lives has now stopped.

As the positive symptoms wane, so can the intensity of care. Since the NHS and Community Care Act started in 1993 all patients admitted to psychiatric hospital must have specially tailored programmes of care that continue until they have recovered (p. 277). For people with acute, transient problems that keep them in hospital for only a few days or weeks, care programmes can be simple and short-lived. But for people with schizophrenia, three-quarters of whom will be left with some kind of illness and disability after their first attacks, care programmes must be wide reaching and durable. Such programmes should spell out details of treatment, names of key staff, practical support, and plans for the future.

Day to day decisions about care are taken between ward doctors and nurses, relatives and – as much as symptoms allow – patients. General progress and bigger decisions about the treatment and care programme are discussed with the consultant psychiatrist at the weekly ward meeting.

In the early stages of treatment most decisions about drugs are the responsibility of doctors, particularly when patients are so ill that they have to have compulsory treatment under the Mental Health Act (see Chapter 9). In England and Wales the treating doctor has sole charge for only the first three months of a compulsory treatment order. After that, any patient who continues to refuse treatment must be seen by an independent doctor appointed by the Mental Health Act Commission, who may also say that treatment must continue. If the treatment order is not renewed after six months, any further treatment is given only with the patient's consent. At this point, or right from the start in the case of patients voluntarily taking treatment, decisions should be negotiated between patient and doctor.

Recovering patients do not need to be supervised closely, as long as they show no signs of harming themselves or others. They can spend more time away from the ward and start to go out, perhaps to shops, with other patients and staff. Later, short visits home can be expanded to last whole weekends and time at home can, increasingly, be spent more actively.

Most sufferers will need some kind of specialized support after discharge from hospital. At the very least, they should be seen regularly by a doctor or community nurse to check their progress and discuss continuing problems. Counselling and help with social welfare problems may be needed by sufferers and their carers. Some patients will not have homes they can return to, perhaps because they were homeless or have become so during many months in hospital, or because the illness has left them unable to cope without special residential care (pp. xxxv–xxxviii).

Such intensive support is most often needed by those patients (about a quarter of sufferers from first attacks) who develop the chronic, negative type of schizophrenia with apathy, loss of interest in life, and lack of emotion (see p. 106). Gradual reintroduction to social activity and ordinary daily tasks through a rehabilitation programme, leading to specialist residential care is the best form of help in this situation. Drugs do not have much effect on negative symptoms. Doses of antipsychotics should be kept as low as possible, keeping the positive symptoms at bay while avoiding sedation. Antidepressants should be considered if there is clear evidence of depression.

Psychological treatments may help people with chronic schizophrenia, particularly in coping with auditory hallucinations. Specific techniques can be taught – distraction (with physical or mental exercises), ignoring, selective listening (only taking notice when the voices say something positive), and setting limits (allocating a certain time of day for listening to the voices). Four sufferers described by researchers in The Netherlands benefited from such techniques.[9] One of their stories is outlined here:

A 42-year-old housewife had been hearing one voice for five years. She had been diagnosed as suffering from schizophrenia and had been admitted four times following suicide attempts ordered by her voice. Eventually she discussed the voice with her husband. He compared the voice with that of a nagging neighbour and asked her if she would harm herself if this neighbour ordered her to do so. Since then, whenever the voice gives the orders, she ignores them. For instance, when she is peeling potatoes and is ordered to stab herself with the knife, she stabs a potato instead. Her control over the voice has increased dramatically and she has not been readmitted since.

Such techniques may not work for everyone: this study was of a small number of people who volunteered to take part in a Dutch national survey about hallucinations. They may not be representative of all people who hear voices.

But many other studies show that sufferers can reduce voices by a variety of methods, including wearing an earplug in one ear, listening to music or other sounds on a personal stereo, and closing the eyes (see Box 7). The effect of shutting out external noise with earplugs and headphones is surprising, given that scientists believe auditory hallucinations to come from inside the head, not through the ears. Presumably the part of the brain that perceives sound, which is thought to function abnormally in schizophrenia, is distracted from picking up the unreal voices.

BOX 7

Ways that sufferers try to reduce auditory hallucinations (voices)

- Wearing an earplug
- Listening to a personal stereo
- Changing posture (lying down, walking)
- Increasing or decreasing contact with other people
- Altering dose of medication
- Distraction from the voices

- Ignoring the voices
- Listening to them selectively
- Setting limits on the voices

Behaviour therapy is sometimes used for people with chronic schizophrenia, as part of a rehabilitation programme. The idea is to encourage normal behaviour and discourage the strange behaviour that can make life outside hospital and acceptance by society so difficult. Following a contract agreed between a patient and staff, normal and socially acceptable behaviour is encouraged by rewarding it, for example with some activity that the person enjoys. Tokens, such as plastic counters, may be used, saved up, and exchanged for rewards. This behaviour modification therapy, as it is called, can help to improve sufferers' social skills and can reduce abnormal behaviour such as shouting back at voices. But withholding certain amenities – watching television, playing snooker, going out for a walk – until they are earned may be unethical. Thus, staff have to be very careful about the kind of rewards used and have to ensure that patients clearly understand and consent to the contracts. Paradoxically, people who are well enough to understand and agree to such contracts are not usually those who most need help to behave normally.

A similar problem affects one small group of people with schizophrenia: those who do not keep up with medication and care outside hospital and tend to relapse frequently, leading to regular emergency readmissions. They are sometimes said to be 'revolving door' patients, stuck in a constant cycle of discharges and readmissions. In the past most would probably have spent their lives in long-stay wards. Now, with antipsychotic drugs and a system of community care it is unjustifiable to keep such patients in hospital once they have recovered from their acute attacks. Community supervision orders, which would be added to Britain's mental health laws, could be imposed on these sufferers to make them comply with the care provided (see Chapter 9). Advocates argue that leaving ill people without care until they become seriously disturbed is just as much an infringement of civil liberties as being forced to accept help.

Avoiding Relapse

CONTINUING TREATMENT

About a quarter of people recover completely from first schizophrenic attacks and never have the illness again. But most sufferers are faced with the prospect of a life-long relapsing illness. For them the most effective way to avoid or delay relapse is careful use of medication, and for many that means continuing antipsychotic drugs indefinitely.

Ideally, a decision to continue or stop treatment should be made on the basis of the patient and his or her family understanding the attendant risks and benefits. Such decisions are, of course, down to individuals but there are a few general issues to consider. Research has shown that medication continued for up to one year after recovery reduces the risk of recurrence, particularly if the sufferer lives in a stressful situation. After a year it is reasonable to reduce the dose of medication gradually and stop it, provided that there are regular checkups. The next attack may not come for many years, but at the first signs of relapse drugs should be restarted. If cessation of treatment is followed quickly by second and subsequent attacks drugs should probably be taken indefinitely.

The prospect of being on medication for ever is hard to accept, particularly for those who become ill in teenage and young adulthood. This is a prospect shared by other young people with life-long illnesses such as diabetes and epilepsy. Doctors and nurses should listen sympathetically to these problems, and work with them. Insisting on the need for medication without sympathizing and without explaining clearly why drugs are so important is unhelpful. So is being critical and angry when sufferers who are undoubtedly at risk of relapse stop treatment suddenly, against advice.

AVOIDING FAMILY STRESS

There is no doubt that living with a person recovering from schizophrenia can be extremely stressful for relatives and other carers. When asked, carers most often complain about the sufferers' strange and unpredictable behaviour, hostility, and poor personal habits. They also complain of disruption in family routines, relationships, and finances. This burden is reflected in carers' poor health. Typically, relatives suffer stress-related symptoms that peak in the first few months after sufferers return home.

Research has shown that the atmosphere in the family can have a profound effect on the risk of schizophrenic relapse. The best atmosphere is of low key support without much overt expression of emotion towards the sufferer. This is dif-ficult to achieve. Some relatives find it hard to resist strong desires to give the sick person a lot of love and attention and practical care; others want to express their frustration and exasperation at putting up with antisocial behaviour. But overcoming these natural desires is worthwhile, because over involvement with and criticism of sufferers by the people they live with have been shown repeatedly to be the two emotional factors that most frequently lead to relapse. Families who act in this way are described by researchers as having a high level of expressed emotion.

The finding that too much emotional contact was bad for people with schizophrenia was made accidentally in the late 1950s by British researchers who were following up men discharged from psychiatric hospital. They found, unexpectedly, that men who went home to live with parents or spouses did less well than men with otherwise similar treatment and prognoses who went to other accommodation or had regular day care. The researchers also found that this effect depended on the amount of contact between the men and their relatives; those having the closest contact relapsed more quickly than the rest. Later research on the nature and quality of contact established a link between relapse and criticism, hostility, and overinvolvement.

Laboratory tests on sufferers have shown that they respond to these kinds of emotional expression by becoming aroused. Because schizophrenia prevents them from expressing this response in the normal way, through their own emotions, sufferers become physically aroused (with extra electrical activity detectable in the skin, raised pulse, and raised blood pressure). Similar overstimulation of the brain is thought to lead to relapse.

Worldwide research on expressed emotion has supported the theory about families and relapse, except in developing countries. A study comparing schizophrenia in families in India and Britain suggested that the more laid back and generally supportive nature of Indian extended families was healthier for people with schizophrenia; perhaps this explains why the disorder is less common in India in the first place.

Thus, families and other carers can help by letting schizophrenic sufferers have as much personal space and independence as possible, while providing a generally supportive environment. This may mean putting up with strange but bearable habits, rather than trying to make sufferers from schizophrenia behave normally all the time. Families with severe problems may be able to be referred to one of the few specialist centres in Britain that offer families education and help to reduce expressed emotion. These centres can also introduce similar families for mutual support.

Families should also encourage and facilitate attendance at day centres and day hospitals for people with schizophrenia. Day care provides activities like those that helped recovery in hospital and, as well as its specific benefits, such care offers time away from the family.

All these aspects of treatment – continuing medication, family support, and day care – should be available to some degree to all people with schizophrenia. But not everyone needs each form of help, and the overall programme of care for someone with schizophrenia must arise from an individual assessment of needs. Box 8 shows where to get further information on schizophrenia.

BOX 8

Further Information on Schizophrenia

The following organizations offer advice and support to sufferers and relatives:
National Schizophrenia Fellowship

Schizophrenia Association of Great Britain

SANE (Schizophrenia – A National Emergency)

MIND

The following books may help too:

The Reality of Schizophrenia by Gwen Howe (Faber and Faber, 1991)

Schizophrenia: Voices in the Dark by Mary Moate and David Enoch (Kingsway Publications, 1990)

Coping with Schizophrenia by Jacqueline M. Atkinson (Thorsons, 1989, 2nd edition)

Living with Schizophrenia by Brenda Lintner (Macdonald Optima, 1989)

Working in Partnership by Liz Kuipers and Paul Bebbington (Heinemann, 1990)

4 DEMENTIAS AND RELATED PROBLEMS

Growing Old, Growing Confused

> All men are mortal: they reflect upon this fact. A great many become old: almost none ever foresees this state before it is upon him. Nothing should be more expected than old age: nothing is more unforeseen.
> From *Old Age* by Simone de Beauvoir[1]

Mental health problems are a common accompaniment to growing old. This is partly because several factors that are known to cause problems like depression – physical ill health, inactivity, isolation, bereavement, and poverty – happen to many old people. And as the brain ages it works less well, like most of the body. Performance in intelligence tests tends to fall with age, and declines fairly steeply after 65. Speed of thinking, problem solving, and capacity to remember recent events may all be reduced.

But IQ tests were designed for use among school children, so they do not measure aspects of intelligence which emerge in adult life, like the ability to make responsible judgments. And it is difficult to compare the performance of young people with today's elderly population who may have had poorer education and poorer nutrition in childhood. Thirdly, any representative sample of old people whose intelligence tests might be used as a norm could include some with early undiagnosed dementia. This would bias the results and lower the average performance on the tests.

Not all elderly people lose their mental faculties, and intellectual deterioration is not an inevitable consequence of growing old. And anyway, for many people the decline in mental sharpness in old age is more than made up for by positive psychological developments. Old age brings an acceptance of life, an ability to see what is important, and an integration of experience that allows people to accept their inevitable mortality.

About a quarter of the very old population does, however, suffer severe deterioration in intellect, health, and independence in the form of what doctors call organic mental illnesses. (In medical jargon organic usually means that something results from structural changes in an organ.) Organic mental illnesses can occur at any age, but are particularly common in old age. They include chronic (which means long-term) illnesses – dementias – as well as acute (transient) states of mental confusion.

Dementias, of which the commonest type is Alzheimer's disease, are responsible for a great deal of disease and disability. They are incurable, progressive, and eventually fatal. Although psychiatry cannot yet do much to prevent or treat these illnesses, psychiatric services help many sufferers and their carers to cope more easily.

Acute confusional states, sometimes called delirium, are short-lived complications of infection and other generalized illnesses. They can occur at any age but the older brain, especially one already damaged by dementia, is particularly susceptible to them.

ACUTE CONFUSIONAL STATES

These are episodes of disorientation, muddled thinking, and disturbed behaviour that start suddenly and do not usually last more than a few days. These symptoms are the external signs of disrupted brain activity caused by reactions to drugs (particularly among elderly people who are usually particularly sensitive to the effects of prescribed drugs), generalized illness – including infection; lack of oxygen; altered blood sugar; and failure of heart, kidney, or liver – and local problems in the brain like stroke, meningitis, or head injury (see Box 1).

BOX 1

> **Main causes of acute confusional states**
>
> Side effects of prescribed drugs
>
> Infections, especially with fever
>
> Interrupted blood supply to brain
>
> Stroke
>
> Heart attack
>
> Lack of oxygen in the blood
>
> Acute chest disease, e.g. pneumonia
>
> Acute heart disease, e.g. heart failure
>
> Toxic chemicals made by tumours (cancers)
>
> Disturbed metabolism
>
> Diabetes complications
>
> Kidney failure

Jack's symptoms were typical of acute confusion:

Jack, 74, was admitted to hospital with pneumonia complicating his chronic bronchitis. He had become mentally confused over the past few days. He was sometimes drowsy, at other times frightened. He called out his wife's name, apparently thinking he was still at home. And, although he recognized her when she came to visit, he became vague and unsure who she was while they talked.

At night Jack became more muddled and afraid, saying there were frightening faces in the darkened room. He kept pulling off the oxygen mask that he needed for his poor breathing, and every so often he would try to get out of bed. Leaving a low light on settled Jack a little, as did firm but calm reassurance from the nurses.

Eventually the antibiotics cleared up Jack's chest infection and associated septicaemia (infection in the blood). As his recovering lungs became more able to collect oxygen, his mind cleared. Jack could not, however, remember much about his stay in hospital.

Lack of oxygen to the brain is a very common cause of acute confusion, and Jack had many of the typical symptoms. His confusion started suddenly and worsened rapidly with his pneumonia. The intensity of his confusion varied and he had some lucid intervals. At other times he did not know where he was, what time it was, or who people were. He drifted in and out of drowsiness during the day, while at night his sleep was erratic. Jack's disorientation was worse at night. He was less able to see and sense his surroundings in the dark and his sense of reality was disrupted by frightening visual hallucinations. All Jack's symptoms stopped when the underlying cause, acute infection, was removed.

As in Jack's case, treatment of acute confusional states mainly involves treating the underlying cause. But the symptoms of acute confusion may be so bad that they need treatment too.

Treating Symptoms of Acute Confusion
Firstly, the sufferer's environment should be made as quiet, reassuring, and constant as possible with the minimum of coming and going. Carers and visitors can help orientation by saying who they are, calling the sufferer by name, and trying to mention the time of day and day of the week in conversation. A soft light left on at night also improves orientation and reduces the likelihood of hallucinations.

If these simple measures are not enough to calm down a very disturbed, confused person, sedatives will help. Small doses of antipsychotic drugs like thioridazine (trade name Melleril), promazine (Sparine), or chlorpromazine (Largactil) are effective and will not cause withdrawal problems.

CHRONIC ORGANIC MENTAL ILLNESSES: DEMENTIAS

> I could see him looking through one of the spy-holes and then he finally opened the door a crack while it was still chained. He did not appear to recognize me and was very suspicious. I just kept talking and eventually he let me in . . . The room was in a chaotic state, the bed was unmade and the sheets were filthy . . . He sat down and kept talking in a distracted way and looking at me with a puzzled expression but without recognition . . . I could not believe that this sad and mad old man was really my husband and the person of whom I had been so afraid. I knew so little about this sort of illness, despite the fact that I was a trained medical practitioner and had even done some psychiatry. At last I realized that his mind was dementing.
>
> From *Alzheimer's Disease: The Long Bereavement* by Elizabeth Forsythe[2]

Britain, like many developed countries, is facing a rising tide of dementia. Around one in ten people over 65 have some symptoms of dementia. This rises to one in four over 85. By the year 2000 the number of people over 65 in Britain will have risen from 8.4 million in 1985 to 9 million, and most of this rise will be accounted for by people over 85. The percentage of the British population with dementia will, therefore, increase; and many sufferers will be looked after by offspring who are also pensioners.

Symptoms of Dementia

Dementia is a progressive state of chronic confusion with intellectual and other types of mental deterioration that end in death. There are several kinds of dementia, all sharing the same general features as described below (see Box 2 for summary).

BOX 2

General features of dementia

Loss of short-term memory

- Forgetting recent events
- Repeating oneself many times without realizing it
- Misplacing things
- Wandering and getting lost

Personality change

Loss of abstract thinking

General psychiatric symptoms

- Loss of reality sense
- Loss of insight
- Delusions
- Hallucinations
- Depression
- Agitation and anxiety
- Disinhibition

Loss of practical mental skills

- Speech problems
- Loss of spatial sense
- Loss of simple practical skills

Physical disability and illness

- Unsteadiness and walking problems
- Incontinence

Loss of independence

- Inability to manage personal affairs
- Poor self-care skills
- Need for continuous care

Loss of Short-Term Memory

Short-term memory is severely affected; remembering what happened earlier that day or even a few minutes ago becomes impossible. But long-term memories of youth and early family life are preserved until the late stages of dementia: Peggy, a woman with dementia, could remember names of school-friends and songs learnt as a child, but she always forgot the name of her regular home help whom she saw three times every week.

Personality Change

Features of personality become coarsened. It loses its individuality, so much so that relatives say things like 'we lost him years before he died.' And personality tends to change for the worst: one of the common first signs of dementia is the development of uncharacteristic selfishness, rudeness, stubbornness, demands for attention, and resistance to other people's ideas and wishes.

As memory continues to fail, sufferers forget who they are, and the last shreds of individuality and personality are lost.

Loss of Abstract Thinking

Thinking becomes less expansive and abstract and more wooden (or, as doctors say, concrete). Sufferers have little conversation. Their interest in the lives of family and friends and in current affairs dwindles until sufferers seem to think about almost nothing except their immediate needs. Albert, a former scientist, came to spend all his waking hours in his armchair, where he would only communicate when he needed to go to the lavatory.

General Psychiatric Symptoms

As well as general intellectual deterioration dementia can include many symptoms seen in other mental illnesses. Grasp on reality is gradually lost and delusions and hallucinations can occur. Delusions are often paranoid: for instance sufferers are convinced that mislaid objects have been stolen by non-existent intruders or other persecutors.

Dementia sufferers often misidentify people and the context in which they meet them. They wrongly identify family members, talk to people on television as if they are in the room and able to hear, fail to recognize their own reflection in a mirror, or say that there are new people in the house when there are not.

Depression and anxiety, often with agitation, are also fairly common among demented people, particularly in the early stages of illness when sufferers still have some insight into what is happening to them. Perhaps the only compensation for the tragedy of Alzheimer's disease is that insight, realizing that one is ill, disappears quite quickly.

Stranger psychiatric symptoms include gross overreactions to events and surroundings, outbursts of disturbed and noisy behaviour, binge eating, and loss of social inhibitions – sometimes resulting in unusually amorous behaviour. These last symptoms are all forms of disinhibition. This occurs most often in types of dementia that particularly affect the brain's frontal lobes, which normally control personality and social behaviour. Disinhibited behaviour can be very difficult for carers to cope with and can make going out or having visitors embarrassing and stressful, especially if the demented person is sexually disinhibited.

Loss of Practical Mental Skills
Abnormalities in more practical brain functions include problems with speech, spatial sense (knowing where things are), and ability to perform simple tasks like dressing or making a cup of tea. Speech may become slurred or strangely muddled – sufferers may lose the ability to name objects correctly, jumble their words, and say certain phrases over and over again. The ability to judge the relative positions of things may be lost; for instance a sufferer may not be able to put a cup on a table without dropping it over the edge. And they can no longer work out how to do things; they may try to dress but end up with clothes on back to front.

Physical Disability and Illness
Finally, the brain damage in dementia becomes so widespread that it affects walking and balance, continence and, in the terminal stage, vital functions like the control of breathing and heartbeat.

Loss of Independence
All of these symptoms of dementia render sufferers increasingly unable to look after themselves. At first practical things like money management, shopping, cooking, and laundry become too difficult. Eventually ordinary self-care is affected. Sufferers need help with even the most basic tasks like washing and dressing. For most this means continuous care by spouses, children, and other relatives; for others it means institutional care or, at the very least, community care. Beatrice, whose story is described here, eventually needed nursing care at home:

> Beatrice, an 83-year-old woman, had had partial blindness for five years as a complication of her diabetes. She used to be sociable, intelligent, and active. But Beatrice's poor vision made going out difficult and she was increasingly confined to her home, where she lived with her 86-year-old husband.
>
> Over the past year Beatrice had become forgetful. On one occasion she went out to the shops and, forgetting where she was going, lost her way home. She was brought back by the police who had found her wandering in streets only 10 minutes away from home.
>
> Beatrice began to live in the past more and more. Her conversation revolved around old memories. She sometimes talked of her long dead parents as if they were still alive, and would say incongruous things about her current job as if she was still a young working woman.
>
> Eventually Beatrice needed help from her husband with washing, dressing and using the toilet because she could not remember or work out what needed doing.

But he had bad arthritis and was quite disabled. He did his best to manage alone, but when he could no longer help Beatrice in and out of the bath he went to their GP for help.

The doctor came to see Beatrice and realized what was happening. She arranged for a district nurse to lift, wash, and dress Beatrice and get her in and out of bed at each end of the day. She also called in a community psychiatric nurse to advise Beatrice's husband on ways of coping and to give him some moral support.

A good account of the way dementia develops and the way it causes forgetfulness, loss of independence, and difficult behaviour was put together by a group of researchers in Cambridge who studied 120 people with dementia and asked those relatives in closest contact with the sufferers about problems that arose from the illness.[3]

The relatives explained how the first signs of dementia appeared, before a clear diagnosis could be made. Sufferers gradually became forgetful and lost interest in doing anything. They were often bad tempered. They would sit and look vague for long periods and not do much else. Relatives started to worry about sufferer's safety outside the home, fearing that they might lose themselves in the town.

As the illness progressed the inactivity and forgetfulness became more and more obvious. Sufferers increasingly needed help with all aspects of daily life: without help they became dishevelled, unsteady on their feet and likely to fall, increasingly immobile, and sometimes incontinent of both urine and faeces. Frequent temper tantrums and demanding behaviour were particularly hard for relatives to cope with; some also had to deal with noisy outbursts and aggressive behaviour.

Eventually, in the final stages of the illness, the biggest strain on relatives was the need for 24-hour care: '[they] cannot be left alone for an hour'. Incontinence was coped with very well: although four-fifths of the most severely demented people were sometimes incontinent, fewer than a quarter of their relatives saw this as a major problem. The second greatest strain was having to cope with noisy disturbed behaviour. Sufferers' increasing inactivity was coped with remarkably well by relatives, perhaps not surprisingly, since it gave them much needed breaks from the burden of care.

Types and Causes of Dementia

The commonest forms of dementia are Alzheimer's disease and multi-infarct dementia. They nearly always affect elderly people, so are sometimes called senile (old age) dementias. About half of all elderly demented people have Alzheimer's disease, about a quarter have multi-infarct dementia, and the rest have a mixture of the two or one of the much rarer dementias.

These other dementias include alcoholic dementia, dementias due to pressure in the brain from hydrocephalus and tumours, Huntington's disease, Pick's disease, Creutz-feld-Jakob disease, and AIDS dementia – all of which usually start before old age. Because of this they are sometimes called presenile dementias. Alzheimer's disease occasionally starts in middle age, too – around one in a thousand of the general population under 65 has the disease. Box 3 summarizes the main types of dementia.

BOX 3

> **Types of dementia**
>
> Senile (old age) dementias
>
> > Alzheimer's disease
> >
> > Multi-infarct dementia
>
> Presenile dementias
>
> > Alzheimer's disease
> >
> > Alcoholic dementia
> >
> > Dementias caused by pressure in the brain
> >
> > > from hydrocephalus
> > >
> > > from tumours and other swellings

Huntington's disease

Pick's disease

Creutzfeld-Jakob disease

AIDS dementia

Senile Dementias

ALZHEIMER'S DISEASE

Alzheimer's disease, named after the physician who first described the characteristic symptoms, was initially thought to affect mainly middle-aged people. It was, therefore, considered to be a purely presenile dementia. But doctors eventually realized that at least half of all senile dementia was also due to Alzheimer's disease, and that the presenile and senile forms were identical.

The main characteristic of Alzheimer's disease is its progressive and relentless course. It usually starts slowly with insidious memory loss. Widespread deterioration in mental functioning follows quickly, leading to death within eight or so years. In the terminal stages of the disease fits sometimes occur.

When Alzheimer's disease starts late, in the 80s or 90s, it is often much more benign. Memory loss remains the most prominent symptom and death from other common causes may occur before the onset of severe disability.

Possible causes of Alzheimer's disease   If the brains of Alzheimer sufferers are examined after death they show several abnormalities whose causes are not fully understood. Overall, the brains are small and shrunken because the disease has killed off many brain cells or neurones. Cell death mainly occurs in the outer layers of the brain, in the part called the cortex, where mental functions like thought, intellect, personality, and the senses are based. Within the brain the ventricles, spaces that contain cerebrospinal fluid, are enlarged. These overall changes are easily visible on brain scans done during life.

Under the microscope the brain tissues contain two abnormal features: plaques containing a protein called amyloid and tangles of small filament-like structures. Both plaques and tangles contain high concentrations of salts that, in turn, contain aluminium. Another widespread chemical change in Alzheimer's disease is a reduction in the chemical messenger acetylcholine in the parts of the brain responsible for intellect and memory. In theory, drugs which raise the level of acetylcholine in the brain could cure or at least slow down the disease.

What causes this brain damage is still not completely clear.[4] What information there is has come mainly from studies of people who develop presenile Alzheimer's disease, before they reach 65. They have more aggressive illnesses with widespread disruption of brain structure and chemistry. And they usually have postmortems, unlike a lot of elderly people who die, so their brains tend to be studied closely.

Other research on people with presenile Alzheimer's disease shows that about one in three has a close relative who also has the disease. This suggests that the cause is at least partly inherited. This is backed up by studies on twins with the disease – identical twins of sufferers are twice as likely to also have it as are non-identical twins, who are genetically just ordinary siblings who happened to get conceived at the same time.

Another intriguing clue to the genetic story is that people with Down's syndrome, a common form of learning disability (mental handicap), invariably develop Alzheimer's disease if they live beyond about 35. And Alzheimer's disease is unusually common among relatives of people with Down's syndrome. Down's syndrome is caused by having an extra chromosome – instead of the normal 23 pairs of human chromosomes (which are strands of genes within the nucleus of every cells) those with this syndrome have three copies of chromosome number 21. Scientists think, therefore, that the basic fault in those cases of Alzheimer's disease that occur in people with Down's syndrome and their families arises from a problem in one or more genes on chromosome 21. The current theory is that amyloid (the protein found in the brain plaques) is produced abnormally by this genetic fault.

But this does not explain why presenile Alzheimer's disease should occur in other families, which it sometimes does. According to sophisticated genetic research done in 1992, these other inherited cases seem to be caused by another genetic abnormality, this time somewhere on chromosome 14.[5] This work on chromosome 14 is just one of many results from the huge international Human Genome Project, which is gradually producing a map of all human chromosomes and unlocking many, many secrets about heredity and disease.

No one is sure, however, what these two genetic findings mean for most people with Alzheimer's disease, who get the disease in old age and do not obviously inherit it from anyone. But in 1993 an abnormality of the gene responsible for production of amyloid, on chromosome 19, gave more clues to the cause of these much commoner cases.[6] The gene abnormality was found among more than two-thirds of relatives of people with senile Alzheimer's disease; so it does not explain all the cases but seems to be important in many. More genetic clues will probably be found over the next few years.

Finally, one non-genetic theory about the cause of Alzheimer's disease has had a lot of publicity. Because high levels of aluminium are often found in sufferers' brains some scientists think that the non-familial cases of the disease could be due to aluminium poisoning from saucepans or drinking water supplies. But neurochemists say that the aluminium does not cause the nerve cell damage that is so central to Alzheimer's disease and that its presence in affected brains is just incidental.

Drug treatments for Alzheimer's disease As yet, there is no cure for Alzheimer's disease. Many sufferers are prescribed psychiatric drugs at some time, but most of these are given to treat additional symptoms like disturbed behaviour, restlessness, insomnia, anxiety, and depression. Many treatments specifically for the dementia have been tried with little success, including vasodilator drugs that increase the brain's blood supply and other drugs that increase concentrations of the brain's chemical messengers, particularly the one called acetylcholine.

One drug, however, does seem to improve sufferers' intellectual functioning, delaying the dementia's progress by about 6–12 months. It is called tacrine (full name tetrahydroaminoacridine or THA), and it acts against the enzyme chemical in the brain that breaks down acetylcholine. Thus it indirectly increases the concentration of acetylcholine in brain cells. As explained above, loss of acetylcholine is one of the features of Alzheimer's disease, and may be the chemical basis for the memory loss and intellectual decline. So tacrine ought to be an effective treatment for Alzheimer's disease; and it probably is – but only to a limited extent.

One of the first studies of tacrine, in 1986, showed it to work dramatically well; others have shown it not to work at all. Psychiatrists and researchers differ widely in their confidence about the drug's effects. One group of researchers at London's Institute of Psychiatry, however, argues that tacrine does work and that the studies that showed no effect were not designed properly. This group have performed two major studies of the drug. The latest, on 65 patients with Alzheimer's disease, showed a definite but limited improvement in tests of intellect and memory within as little as two to four weeks, which then stayed at a plateau during treatment but tailed off again when treatment was stopped.[7]

Tacrine does not seem to be a miracle cure that completely reverses Alzheimer's disease to normal: it just seems to slow down the deterioration. Perhaps tacrine will prove useful in staving off symptoms while long-term care is arranged.

MULTI-INFARCT DEMENTIA
This is the second commonest type of dementia in old age, accounting for up to a quarter of all cases. Unlike Alzheimer's disease, it has a reasonably well understood cause.

Multi-infarct dementia arises from a succession of small strokes, each killing off small areas of brain tissues. The medical term infarct means localized death of tissues, and cerebral (or brain) infarction is a medical term for stroke.

The main cause of strokes and of multi-infarct dementia is high blood pressure. Because high blood pressure damages blood vessels, making their walls thick and inelastic, it eventually reduces the blood supply to the body's organs, including the brain. One of the arguments for treating high blood pressure throughout adult life, although it rarely produces any symptoms itself, is to try and prevent strokes. There is no specific treatment for multi-infarct dementia except the control of blood pressure and any other problems that damage blood vessels like diabetes and, of course, smoking.

In many ways multi-infarct dementia is similar to Alzheimer's disease and its end result is the same. But there is one important difference – the course of the illness. The symptoms of multi-infarct dementia develop patchily and intermittently, causing deterioration in clear steps rather than a relentless and continuous decline. The severity of the forgetfulness and disorientation may vary from day to day or even over a few hours, and are often worse at night. In this way the symptoms are like those of acute confusional states, which were described on p. 133. Underlying these ups and downs, however, is a very gradual overall deterioration.

People with multi-infarct dementia often understand what is happening to them, because the parts of the brain responsible for grasp on reality and insight are affected quite late in the disease. Understandably, this makes many sufferers depressed or anxious. Others get irritable and angry, particularly when trying to do something that has become difficult as a result of the disease.

Insight is not the only reason for sufferers to have mood problems. Some also seem to lose control over the expression of emotions, perhaps because the part of the brain that controls emotions is damaged. Sufferers have strange and virtually unprompted outbursts of laughing or crying, for instance when someone walks into the room. This problem, which is usually more distressing for carers than for sufferers, is sometimes given the unpleasant but graphic name 'emotional incontinence'.

Harry had multi-infarct dementia:

> Harry was 73 when he collapsed and lost consciousness for several hours. When he came round in hospital he had lost the use of the muscles of one arm and one side of his face. Harry had had a stroke. He was confused for a few days but recovered and was sent home with support from a district nurse and a physiotherapist.
>
> Over the next few months Harry's muscle power slowly came back. During the following year he had several similar, though milder attacks of transient muscle weakness. He never seemed quite the same afterwards. Gradually, in steps, Harry was losing his memory and intellectual abilities.
>
> Harry began to get depressed, so his GP put him on some antidepressant tablets. He was already on blood pressure tablets. On top of his generally low mood, which improved only slightly with treatment, he had uncontrollable and unexplained episodes of crying and laughing.
>
> Over the next three years Harry lost interest in what his children and grandchildren were doing. His wife needed more and more support and help in looking after him. By the time he had deteriorated enough to need almost constant care, his wife had made the hard decision to find a nursing home for him. But before she made any arrangements, Harry died of another stroke.

Presenile Dementias

Alzheimer's disease is the commonest cause of both senile and presenile dementias. It probably accounts for at least 65% of all presenile dementias. Multi-infarct and alcoholic each account for about 10%, dementias due to pressure in the brain for about 5% each, Huntington's disease for about 3%, and the other, very rare, dementias shown in Box 3 make up the rest.

ALCOHOLIC DEMENTIA

Heavy drinking over many years kills brain cells and makes the brain shrink. Up to two-thirds of heavy drinkers are thought to develop at least a degree of this progressive dementia eventually. Given that too much alcohol is a common cause of high blood pressure, multi-infarct dementia often affects heavy drinkers too. When both types occur together there is a continuous deterioration punctuated by stepwise decline.

The other long-term dementia-like state that can affect heavy drinkers is Korsakoff's disease (see p. 178). This is caused by lack of a B vitamin called thiamine, and it is sometimes at least partly reversible if thiamine is given.

DEMENTIA CAUSED BY PRESSURE IN THE BRAIN

The brain is bathed by cerebrospinal fluid which circulates through it in a network of canals and spaces called ventricles. When this network becomes blocked, in a condition called hydrocephalus (water on the brain), the fluid's pressure increases and squashes the brain. If this increase in pressure occurs very gradually it may not be obvious until it has already killed many brain cells. When this dementia develops in old age it may be, quite reasonably, assumed to be due to Alzheimer's disease or multiple infarcts. The real diagnosis will be made only by performing tests like brain scans.

Other forms of swelling in the brain can also compress and damage brain cells. These swellings may be tumours or abscesses and other sites of infection – for instance in tuberculosis.

If these causes of increased pressure are found in time and treated the dementia may be at least partly reversed.

HUNTINGTON'S DISEASE

This is a serious hereditary disease which affects around 2500 people at any time in the UK. It is caused by a dominant gene, which means that children of sufferers have a fifty-fifty chance of also getting it. And people with the faulty gene always develop the disease. Tragically, they do not usually do so until their 30s and 40s, after most of them will have had children and already passed on the gene.

Huntington's disease starts either with strange movements or with psychological problems like depression, or both. The movement disorder, or chorea, consists of repetitive movements of the head and limbs. These may be no more than facial tics and exaggerated foot tapping at first. Eventually, over several years, widespread and persistently abnormal movements develop, making walking difficult and causing considerable disability.

Along with these movement problems goes a slowly progressive dementia. Insight is often retained in the first few years and, understandably, this can lead to anger and distress when symptoms occur. Mercifully, insight is lost as the dementia progresses and irritability is replaced by apathy or calm.

The gene for Huntington's disease has been identified. This means that young people with relatives who suffer from the disease can take a test to see whether they have the gene too. Anyone wanting a test should be given sensitive counselling beforehand, explaining the disease and discussing all the implications of a positive result.

PICK'S DISEASE

The cause of Pick's disease is not known, but some evidence suggests that is probably another partially hereditary dementia. It mainly destroys cells in the frontal lobes of the brain where personality and intellect, but not memory, are based. In the late stages of the disease it affects the temporal lobes at the side of the brain, leading to jumbled and repetitive speech and severe narrowing of vocabulary. Pick's disease is not treatable and usually leads to death within about 10 years.

Tragically, Pick's disease can start at any age from the early 20s. But it appears most commonly in the 40s and 50s. The first sign of Pick's disease is usually a persistent change in personality.

For example, one 28-year-old woman who was previously very houseproud suddenly became apathetic and disinterested in her household when she was 34 weeks pregnant with her second child. Tiredness, depression, and even schizophrenia were all diagnosed over the next year as she became extremely moody and at times very odd. Then she developed speech problems and some abnormal muscle reflexes. A brain scan showed shrinkage of the frontal and temporal lobes of her brain and Pick's disease was diagnosed. Within two years of the disease's onset the woman was living in a long-stay ward, and was extremely disturbed.[8]

CREUTZFELD-JAKOB DISEASE
This is a very rare, rapidly progressive dementia usually resulting in death within two years. Under the microscope after death an affected brain appears pitted with small holes like a sponge.

The disease is thought to be caused by infection with a small virus-like particle called a prion. It can only be passed on within nerve tissue, other tissues that contain nerves, and substances derived from nerve tissue. Some sufferers have caught this disease from corneal transplants given to restore sight after the removal of cataracts. Other people have caught Creutzfeld-Jakob disease from a hormone preparation that they were given to treat dwarfism during late childhood – the growth hormone was extracted from the pituitary glands of dead people's brains. In both cases sufferers were unlucky enough to receive samples from people who had died of Creutzfeld-Jakob disease, unbeknown to doctors at the time. People close to known sufferers are advised not to come into contact with body fluids, although the risk of infection through such ordinary contact is probably very low.

Creutzfeld-Jakob disease is now thought to be one of a group of similar dementias that affect humans and animals. Other examples are the now notorious bovine spongiform encephalopathy (BSE or 'mad cow disease'), scrapie in sheep, and a similar condition in mink. Indeed, BSE seems to have arisen when cattle were given food that included offal and meat from sheep that had scrapie. Whether BSE can be transmitted to man by eating infected meat and meat products (that inevitably contain many nerve cells) is not really settled. The government insists that diseased meat is removed from the food chain before it reaches the market. But some scientists have yet to be convinced that there is no danger to humans.

AIDS DEMENTIA

Acquired human immunodeficiency syndrome (AIDS) is caused by HIV, the human immunodeficiency virus. The main symptoms of AIDS are severe infections and cancers which arise because the body's damaged immune system cannot fight them off. Less well known is the dementia, which eventually affects around 90% of sufferers.

AIDS dementia starts with apathy, social withdrawal, and poor concentration. It progresses to memory loss and widespread mental deterioration. In its terminal stages AIDS dementia can cause complete loss of speech, incontinence, and muscle paralysis.

At least two causes of this dementia are known: brain damage due to direct infection with HIV and damage due to the other infections and cancers that occur in AIDS. Dementia due to HIV is slowly progressive and may be halted or at least delayed by treatment against HIV. Dementia due to the other infections in AIDS can occur suddenly and may be reversed with treatment of those infections.

Health Services for People with Dementia and Their Carers
Although the NHS provides specialized services for people with AIDS, most people with dementia – even young ones – are referred to services for elderly people. This partly reflects the general inability of the NHS to arrange long-term specialized care for very rare problems. It also reflects the practical point that people with dementia need more or less the same kind of care, regardless of age.

Most medical care for elderly people – and anyone else, for

that matter – is provided by GPs. More specialized health care for elderly people with complicated problems is provided by two types of service: old age medicine (also called geriatric medicine) and old age psychiatry (also called psychogeriatrics and psychiatry for the elderly mentally ill). Both specialties provide care that reflects the different ways that common diseases affect elderly people.

Consultant geriatricians are physicians who have specialized in those aspects of internal medicine that relate specifically to old people. These consultants and their teams understand how diseases like strokes, heart disease, chest problems, and diabetes often affect elderly people differently from younger people and they also understand the special problems that disease and disability bring to this age group. Consultant psychogeriatricians, on the other hand, understand that mental illnesses like depression and schizophrenia may have special features in elderly people that make diagnosis hard; and they too understand the practical problems that this age group faces from disease and disability.

Dementia is a physical brain disease that causes both physical and psychiatric symptoms. Not surprisingly, therefore, health care for elderly people with dementia is shared by both geriatric and psychogeriatric disciplines. Ideally, the two specialties work closely together and provide the aspects of care that each is most adept at. In theory, therefore, someone whose dementia was causing considerable immobility and incontinence which had led to a bladder infection and pressure sores on the buttocks would be referred to a geriatrician. And someone else, whose dementia was causing restlessness, wandering, and noisy shouting, would see a psychogeriatrician. Someone with all these problems might receive care from both kinds of specialist, coordinated by the GP. In practice, however, the decision to refer to one or other of the specialties is made by GPs and is often arbitrary or is based on pragmatic factors like which team has the most hospital beds. And, as long as sufferers and their carers get the help they need, the distinction between the two specialties does not really matter. The route to such help, whoever ends up providing it, starts with the GP.

The Role of the General Practitioner

A GP will usually provide the bulk of health care for someone with dementia, at least until severe disease and disability develops. Firstly, they assess sufferers and make a diagnosis. As well as listening to patients' and carers' accounts of the problems so far, this will involve physical and mental state examinations and, more often than not, some tests. Blood tests and X-ray examinations will be done to rule out reversible causes for the symptoms, particularly the diseases that cause acute confusional states (see p. 133). Blood tests to rule out syphilis may also be done; not because the GP suspects that the sufferer led an immoral life, but because syphilis infection was very common a few decades ago and was a cause of much severe mental illness, including dementia.

What happens once the diagnosis of dementia is confirmed depends on the nature of the sufferer's problems. Perhaps the doctor has been called because the elderly person has become too forgetful to buy and cook food regularly and her only daughter works full time and cannot do much to help out during the day. For the time being, practical help from the local social services home care department – meals on wheels and a home help twice a week to do the heavy housework and buy essential groceries – may be all the elderly person needs. At this stage, while the sufferer is happy and safe to live on her own at home, health problems will be dealt with by the GP.

Later, when the dementia has taken hold and started to cause disabling health problems that are beyond the practical scope of the GP and primary care team, or are making living at home unsafe and unsuitable, a specialist will be called in.

The Role of the Specialist

Specialist geriatricians and psychogeriatricians tend to assess referred patients at home, for several reasons. Firstly, this is convenient for sufferers. Secondly, it is often the best way to meet and listen to the carers who spend most time with sufferers and understand better than anyone the nature and extent of the problems caused by the dementia. Lastly, home visits allow doctors to see for themselves the domestic circumstances and to see how well sufferers are coping with everyday life. These important factors are hard to understand when assessment is done in a hospital clinic.

The main assessment usually includes further physical examination, sometimes more tests, and always a mental state examination (see p. xvii). During the mental state examination the doctor will test the sufferer's intellectual abilities and memory, using questions like 'What day is it today?' 'Where are we?' 'Who is the Prime Minister?' Many of these questions may seem too easy or even insulting for many people with early dementia. But they are good at picking up problems that sufferers may have managed to compensate for in other ways, for example by always choosing to talk about old times rather than recent events which have become too hard to remember.

Further assessment may involve other professionals; for instance an occupational therapist may visit to see whether practical aids like handles for the bath or a seat in the shower need installing.

Specialist assessment does not necessarily lead to immediate specialist care. Often the geriatrician or psychogeriatrician simply advises the GP about continuing care. These days services for elderly people have moved away from institutional care, aiming instead to help clients to stay in their own homes for as long as possible. This is one of the keystones of the community care policy that has been developed by successive governments over the past four or five decades. This is probably in line with what most people want, although it implies acceptance of a certain degree of risk to the safety of people on the borderline of coping independently.

Community Care for Elderly People
Community care services have developed gradually since the welfare state was set up nearly 50 years ago. Since

1990, however, they have begun to expand considerably in line with the NHS and Community Care Act of that year.

In essence, the policy states that people whose disabilities and illnesses make them dependent on long-term health and social care should be helped to retain their independence as long as possible (see pp xxxv–xxxviii for more on community care). If all goes to plan, this should mean that people needing such care are carefully assessed and are offered tailored packages of care that are coordinated and budgeted by care managers working in social services, in close consultation with all the relevant health and social care professionals. For elderly people with dementia and, for that matter, any long-term disability or illness that requires extra care, ideal community care has several tiers (see Box 4).

BOX 4

Community care services for elderly people with dementia and other long-term health problems

Home care

- Home helps
- Meals on wheels
- Mental health care – from community psychiatric nurses
- Physical nursing (including bathing) – from district nurses
- Help with practical skills – from occupational therapists
- Befriending for isolated people – from volunteers
- Advice on financial welfare and on all home care services, advocacy (speaking up for those who cannot get what they need) – from social workers

Day care

- Social activities and support – at day centres and lunch clubs
- Assessment and health care – at day hospitals

Respite care

- Temporary residential care, for a week or two, to give carers (and sufferers) a break – at hospitals and nursing homes

Residential care

- Old people's homes
- Nursing homes

Support and advice for carers

- Relatives' groups – at hospitals and residential homes
- Local and national voluntary organizations

Hospital Care for Elderly People

Both geriatric and psychogeriatric services provide a range of hospital care. This includes admission wards and day hospitals where people can be assessed and where fairly intensive help can be given to those who need it but can still live in the community. Long-term care in hospital is reserved for people who need continuous medical and nursing care that cannot be provided at home or in nursing homes. Although dementias are not, on the whole, treatable, medical and nursing care can do much to alleviate suffering.

Help from Voluntary Organizations

Health and social services do not always provide for all the things that sufferers and their carers need. Personal experience, in particular, is something that many self-help and support groups can offer. Talking to someone who really knows what it is like to look after an elderly relative day in and day out can help carers to keep going. Increasingly, voluntary organizations are providing more mainstream care as well, through paid contracts with local authorities and health authorities.

The main voluntary organizations and charities for people with dementia and their carers are listed in Box 5 and their addresses are given in Appendix 2.

BOX 5

Support organizations for people with dementia and their carers

For people with senile dementias

- Age Concern
- Help the Aged
- Alzheimer's Disease Association

For people with presenile dementias

- Huntington's Disease Association
- Terrence Higgins Trust

Specifically for carers

- Carers National Association
- The Relatives' Association

These books may help too:

The 36-Hour Day by N. Mace and P. Robins (Hodder & Stoughton and Age Concern, 1985)

Alzheimer's Disease: The Long Bereavement by Elizabeth Forsythe (Faber & Faber, 1990)

---

5 ALCOHOL AND DRUG PROBLEMS

Holidays in Hell?

Linda got her soma. Thenceforward she remained in her little room on the thirty-seventh floor of Bernard's apartment house, in bed, with the radio and television always on . . . and the soma tablets within reach of her hand – there she remained; and yet wasn't there at all, was all the time away, infinitely far away, on holiday; on holiday in some other world, where the music of the radio was a labyrinth of sonorous colours, a sliding, palpitating labyrinth, that led (by what beautifully inevitable windings) to a bright centre of absolute conviction . . .

From *Brave New World* by Aldous Huxley[1]

USE OF MIND-ALTERING DRUGS

Aldous Huxley's futuristic *Brave New World* could have been perfect. Babies were made and cultured in test tubes and everyone ended up fit and happy to work hard or play hard, depending on their places in the caste system. The state ensured that no one had expectations that were not fulfilled. Yet the brave new people still needed the drug soma, 'a substitute for alcohol and narcotics, something at once less harmful and more pleasure giving than gin or heroin'.

As Huxley explained, 'reality, however utopian, is something from which people feel the need of taking pretty regular holidays . . . the freedom to daydream under the influence of dope and movies and the radio [helps to reconcile subjects] to the servitude which is their fate.' First published in 1932, *Brave New World* would not have rung true if its characters had not had this most basic of human requirements, a recreational drug.

Most societies endorse one or more mind-altering drugs for recreation, religious rites, or for oiling the wheels of everyday life. Socially acceptable drugs are considered beneficial, refreshing, and even sacred. They are distributed by businessmen and used by consumers. Their pleasant effects are emphasized. People who suffer the drugs' adverse effects are considered different and less good or healthy than the rest of society. Socially unacceptable drugs, on the other hand, are dangerous and evil and are distributed by pushers and traffickers. Abusers and addicts are ostracized and punished.

Some drugs used in Western societies have fitted both categories – acceptable and unacceptable – at different times in history. Alcohol, tobacco, caffeine, opium and its opiate products, cocaine, and cannabis have all had their social ups and downs. Tea and coffee, for instance, were fiercely condemned in the *British Medical Journal* in 1890:

> Much has been said concerning the undoubtedly evil effects of excessive tea drinking. Dr F. Mendel has recently [studied] the results of an unbridled abuse of coffee . . . whilst women of the working classes [in England] are often addicted to dosing themselves with tea that has stood too long . . . workmen's wives at Essen drink coffee from morning till night, [resulting in] general weakness, depression of spirits, and an aversion to labour . . . they require rest from work, open air exercise, cold ablutions followed by friction, and small doses of brandy.

Calling tea, coffee and alcohol drugs may seem odd. But it's accurate. The word drug means any substance, whether natural or man-made, which is taken for some specific effect. Drugs with psychological or mind-altering effects have several broad actions: some stimulate and others depress brain activity, some cause hallucinations, and some cause addiction. Many have a mixture of these actions.

Amphetamines, nicotine, caffeine and cocaine increase arousal and alertness. Alcohol, tranquillizers, solvents and opiates like heroin cause an overall depression of brain activity that can be pleasantly intoxicating or relaxing but can also cause depressed mood. Drugs like LSD (lysergic acid dyethylamide) and magic mushrooms alter perception, producing hallucinations. So do dance drugs like ecstasy, which are also stimulants. Cannabis causes hallucinations in big doses, brain depression in small doses. Nicotine, alcohol, opiates and cocaine cause addiction.

People deliberately use drugs to achieve these effects. But not everyone uses them in the same way. Some people, particularly teenagers, experiment with drugs; others use drugs for recreation and fun; others have to use drugs because they have become addicted (see Box 1).

BOX 1	**Properties and modes of use of mind-altering drugs**
	Properties
	• Stimulant
	• Depressant
	• Hallucinogenic
	• Dependence-inducing
	Modes of use
	• Experimental
	• Recreational
	• Dependent

Drug dependence and drug addiction mean the same thing. But addiction has attracted bad connotations over the years and dependence is now the preferred term. People who are dependent on drugs are called users or misusers, less stigmatizing and pejorative words than addict. Whatever words are used, the problem is the same: certain drugs have properties that make people take them repeatedly. The main such property of these drugs is that they cause unpleasant withdrawal syndromes when they are stopped. Withdrawal syndromes include psychological symptoms like craving, irritability, and depression and physical symptoms like shaking, nausea, and stomach upsets. Users soon come to fear these symptoms and try to avoid them. Continuing the drugs keeps the symptoms away. But withdrawal syndromes are not the only reason for continued use; the drugs' pleasant effects and the culture they create also make giving up very hard.

Taking drugs does not always cause problems. Many people use alcohol, tea, coffee, cannabis, and hallucinogens in moderation and in safe ways. But even occasional moderate use can be dangerous in unsafe circumstances – for instance a few drinks can impair concentration and reaction time enough to make driving dangerous.

There are many kinds of drug problem. Most people's image of someone with a drug problem is an HIV positive heroin addict living off prostitution and crime to support a life-threatening habit. But failing to give up cigarettes when you have bronchitis, being unable to go to work unless you have a couple of drinks, and being unable to sleep without a tranquillizer are all drug problems. These problems may seem relatively trivial. But official statistics in the UK show that alcohol intoxication is involved in 65% of suicide attempts, 3 million working days are lost each year through alcohol dependence, and around 175,000 people are dependent on tranquillizers.[2] In an average year alcohol causes 30,000 premature deaths, tobacco causes 100,000, heroin causes 200, solvents 150, amphetamine and ecstasy 2 or 3, and LSD none.[3]

For some people at least, drugs provide harmless breaks from life's problems. But for many these breaks turn out to be holidays in hell.

Causes of Drug Taking

Many factors dictate why people use drugs. Splitting them into personal and social causes makes them easier to describe (see Box 2). In reality, however, drug use arises from a variable mixture of these and other factors.

BOX 2

Causes of drug taking

Personal causes

- Inheritance – gender, family traits
- Age – young people use drugs out of curiosity, rebellion, to deal with anxiety and sexual worries, family stress, alienation
- Fulfilment of needs
- Emotional and mental health problems – personal problems and life events, self-medication, self-destruction, personality problems, depression

Social causes

- Cultural and historical factors
- Availability – certain occupations
- Peer pressure
- Social deprivation – unemployment, lack of education

Personal Causes

INHERITANCE

Heavy drinking and alcohol dependence sometimes run in families.[4] This is not surprising; children often adopt their parents' habits. But there may be at least an element of genetic predisposition to heavy drinking: some children who are born in families with alcohol problems but are brought up elsewhere, away from their own parents' influence, are still prone to alcohol problems themselves. Research in Denmark showed that adopted boys whose natural parents were alcohol dependent were four times more likely than other adopted boys to develop alcohol problems in adult life. Similar findings have been made in adoption studies in the US and Sweden and in twin studies.

There was great excitement in 1990 in the US when newspapers said that the gene for alcoholism had been found. They were referring to research that found a link between alcohol problems and a gene on chromosome 1. But the finding was made in a small number of people and has not been confirmed by subsequent research. In fact more recent research on twins with alcohol problems suggests that genetic inheritance is less important than other factors shared within families like upbringing and general culture.

Even if genes are partly to blame for the development of alcohol problems, no one knows exactly what physical defect may be inherited. It is most likely to be a problem with the enzyme chemicals involved in absorbing and getting rid of alcohol, making some people absorb more alcohol or break down less alcohol per drink than others.

Problems with other drugs do not seem to be inherited.

AGE

The commonest age for experimentation with drugs is adolescence. The Youth Lifestyles Report for 1993 said that nearly a third of 15–24-year-olds surveyed admitted taking drugs, and research in Manchester suggests that two-fifths of 16-year-olds in the North West of England are taking drugs.[5] Teenagers try drugs for many reasons including curiosity, peer pressure and the desire not to be alienated, rebellion, and family troubles. Drugs can also help to ease social anxieties and worries about sex.

FULFILMENT OF BASIC NEEDS

Many psychologists and philosophers believe, like Aldous Huxley, that mankind needs mind-altering experiences to ease the monotony of life. Drug use is just one example; religion, art, and music are others.

Mankind also needs fun. Many people use drugs because they enjoy them.

EMOTIONAL AND MENTAL HEALTH PROBLEMS

Drug misuse often develops gradually from ordinary social use. But some people deliberately increase their drug use because they want to avoid or block out unpleasant feelings. The feelings may be transient, arising from specific personal problems and events. Often, however, the feelings arise from long-term mental health problems like depression, personality disorders, and underlying suicidal urges.

Social Causes

CULTURAL AND HISTORICAL FACTORS

As discussed already, some drugs and their effects are socially acceptable. Patterns of social acceptability and use vary in different countries. For instance, tobacco is mostly smoked in Britain but in Sweden it is widely used as snuff and as pellets that are stuffed under the lip and absorbed through the gums. Patterns vary over time, too. Opium and its derivatives like laudanum were freely on sale from British grocers until 1868 and thereafter from chemists for many years.

AVAILABILITY

Whether people can easily get hold of drugs depends on their culture, their social lives, jobs, and legal restrictions, among many factors. Easy availability tends to increase use, not surprisingly. Anaesthetists, for instance, who have daily access to many dangerous drugs, have a high incidence of drug problems. And publicans are at high risk of getting alcohol problems.

Availability of illegal or 'street' drugs depends on local culture. In some towns most drug users take pills, in others – particularly cities with considerable social deprivation – the biggest problem is of intravenous drug use.

EMPLOYMENT

Given that consumption of alcohol increases with income, it is not surprising that regular heavy drinking is commoner among professionals and managers than among manual workers. This difference is most marked for women: in 1988 government figures showed that 14% of professional women drank more than the recommended safe limit compared with 8% of women in semi-skilled and unskilled jobs.

Unemployment, however, confuses this picture. Most unemployed people in Britain in the 1980s were from manual jobs and, in keeping with the overall findings about income and drinking, they drank less than richer people. But those unemployed people who did drink tended to drink very heavily, particularly in dangerous binges. It is not hard to imagine why.

Treating Drug Problems – General Principles

Whether the drug causing problems is alcohol or heroin, treatment has certain common features (see Box 3).

BOX 3

Treatments for drug problems
Recognize the problem
Quantify the problem
Use information about the problem to cut down or stop drug use
Specific treatment
First aid for intoxication
Drying out
Counselling
Behaviour therapy
Psychotherapy

The first step is realizing that there is a problem. This may seem obvious, but family and friends often notice that things are getting out of hand before the drug user realizes. One reason for this disparity is that recreational or social use may develop very gradually into a problem. And drug users who are used to a social peer group, perhaps drinkers in a pub or friends who smoke cannabis, compare themselves with fellow users and think their own behaviour is normal. Relatives and friends who do not get drunk or stoned, however, may be much more aware of the effects of intoxication and other drug-related behaviour. Even when confronted with other people's view of the problem, users often strongly deny that anything is wrong.

Realization that a drug is causing problems may only come at a time of crisis; when a spouse threatens to leave, a job is on the line, a criminal charge is made, or a physical problem caused by the drug develops. For many people the decision to tackle a drug problem is made only when it can no longer be ignored.

One way that people can start facing up to their drug problems is to find out for themselves the problem's real extent. A good way to start is to record honestly in a diary every drug-taking episode, along with the circumstances and feelings that surrounded it. The results at the end of the first week may be surprising and worrying.

Drawing up a two column list about the drug use helps to clarify what the diary shows up. The list is like a balance sheet of profit and loss. For example, someone worried about their drinking might write in the profit column 'I like the taste. I meet friends when I drink. It makes me more sociable. It makes me forget my problems.' In the loss column would go 'It costs too much. It gives me stomach ache. My boss complains when I'm hungover at work. It makes me argue with my wife. Forgetting problems makes them worse.' A similar list drawn up by a spouse or other close contact may be more brutal and honest.

A simple questionnaire called the CAGE is remarkably accurate at picking up problem drinking (see Box 4). Researchers found that up to three-quarters of people who said yes to at least two of the four questions had alcohol problems, as confirmed by much more detailed interviews.[6]

BOX 4

CAGE questionnaire for problem drinking

Have you ever felt you ought to Cut down your drinking?

Have people Annoyed you by criticizing your drinking?

Have you ever felt bad or Guilty about your drinking?

Have you ever had a drink first thing in the morning (an Eye opener) to steady your nerves or get rid of a hangover?

[The name CAGE comes from the first letters of the key words in the four questions – Cut, Annoyed, Guilty, Eye opener.]

Diaries, lists, and questionnaires like these give a lot of clues about how to cut down the drug use, and they may be enough for some people. Many people, however, will need the help of someone else who knows about drug problems. There are many self-help groups, both locally and nationally, for people with drug problems. Most provide information and support (often for families too), and some provide practical help and treatment. These groups are described in more detail later in this chapter and their addresses are given in Appendix 2.

People wanting professional help can go to a GP or straight to a local community alcohol or drugs team, as long as it accepts self-referrals. Most areas of Britain have such teams, which usually comprise doctors, nurses, psychologists, social workers, and sometimes probation officers. Their contact addresses and phone numbers are available in directories of local services, in health centres, and in social services offices.

Drugs can cause a wide range of problems and there is a correspondingly wide variety of approaches to treatment. Acute intoxication may cause collapse, needing first aid (see Box 5).

BOX 5

First Aid for Intoxication and Collapse

Whether collapse is due to alcohol, ecstasy, solvents, or any other mind-altering drug the basic principles are the same:

Call an ambulance

Check that the collapsed person is breathing and has a heartbeat

If there is no breathing or heartbeat and someone knows how to resuscitate, let them try

If the person is breathing and has a heartbeat put the person in the recovery position (on one side with head tilted back to keep air passages open, and uppermost arm and leg bent to stop the person rolling onto their face)

Try to rouse the person by talking to them

Do not try to make them drink or vomit

Physical complications of drug use may need treatment in hospital, particularly medical emergencies like DTs (delirium tremens, which can occur during alcohol withdrawal) and drugs overdoses. Withdrawal from dependence-inducing drugs can be treated by drying out or detoxification: other drugs are given as safer substitutes and are reduced slowly causing minimal symptoms. Nicotine patches for smokers and methadone for heroin users are two examples of drying out.

Outpatient counselling and group therapies can alter patterns of drug use and help users to achieve agreed targets and goals. Sometimes these therapies deal with the underlying problems that first led to drug use.

These general principles apply to any kind of problem, whether due to alcohol or another drug. More detailed information follows:

ALCOHOL

> We admitted we were powerless over alcohol – that our lives had become unmanageable.
>
> *Step One of the twelve steps that Alcoholics Anonymous asks its members to accept*

Between 6% and 8% of all consumer spending in Britain goes on alcohol, more than is spent on clothes or on running cars. More than a third of this money is collected by the government in excise duty and value added tax. Compared with incomes, alcohol is now relatively cheaper in Britain than at any time since the end of the Second World War. Consumption is higher now than at any time since the early 1900s, at just under 10 litres of pure alcohol a year for each member of the adult population. In 1987, for example, the average adult Briton consumed 235 pints of beer, 21 bottles of wine, 12 pints of cider, and 3 bottles of spirits. And these statistics do not include home-brewed beers.

The amount of harm caused by alcohol is closely related to the average consumption: as the average rises more people drink at harmful levels. Harm is not confined to a small group of people dependent on alcohol; in fact most alcohol problems affect people who for most of their lives drink at only moderately high levels. Medical and social campaigners argue that the burden of alcohol problems could be reduced most easily and quickly by the government, simply by considerably increasing taxes on alcohol.

Defining Alcohol Problems

The amount that people can drink without risking harm varies among individuals and with different patterns of drinking. Indeed, a little alcohol probably does you good. Many studies have shown that people who regularly have one or two drinks a day are less likely to get heart problems and strokes than heavier drinkers or teetotallers.[7] This is probably because a little alcohol increases the concentration of a special form of fat in the blood which, for various reasons, is good for the heart and blood vessels.

But regular drinking above certain levels each week can be dangerous. Comparing numbers of drinks taken is meaningless, because a pint of beer and a glass of sherry contain different amounts of alcohol. The most accurate way to assess intake is to work out the amount of pure alcohol consumed. But this is complicated and technical and means nothing to most drinkers.

So researchers have come up with an easy rule of thumb – the unit of alcohol. One unit of alcohol is contained in one pub measure of spirits, vermouth, port, or sherry; one pub glass of wine, or half a pint of ordinary strength beer or lager. Some drinks contain surprisingly large amounts of alcohol. One pint of average cider contains three units. Strong beers and lagers may contain four units in one 12oz can.

The upper limit of safe drinking for women is around 14 units a week and for men it is 21 units. One in four men and one in twelve women in Britain drink more than these recommended levels. Women's bodies are more sensitive to alcohol than men's and are damaged by lower levels of drinking. Until recently this was explained by women's lower weights and their tendency to have more fat and less water in their bodies than men. Alcohol is carried around the body with water, so it is more diluted in men than in women. Recently, however, scientists have found that women are less able than men to start breaking down alcohol in the stomach before it is absorbed. This is because women have relatively less of an alcohol-destroying enzyme in their stomach linings. Women, therefore, absorb a greater proportion of the alcohol that they drink – even a little can go a long way.

The risks from drinking rise gradually. At weekly levels just above 14 units for women and 21 for men there may be little long-term risk to health. Above 28 units a week the risk of the serious liver disease, cirrhosis, is increased six times. Above 40 units a week the risk is 14 times greater than it is for men who drink only a little. Above 30 units a week men become increasingly likely to die in the next 10 years. At all these levels of drinking, women are assumed to be at considerably greater risk of harm. Summing up, men who drink more than 50 units of alcohol a week (three and a half pints of beer a day) and women who drink more than 35 units a week (less than a bottle of wine a day) are highly likely to suffer a wide range of health problems (see Box 6).

BOX 6	**Safe and unsafe levels of alcohol intake**
	Safe weekly levels • Up to 21 units for men • Up to 14 units for women *Very unsafe weekly levels* • 50 or more units for men • 35 units or more for women

Symptoms of Problem Drinking

During the 1980s alcohol was responsible for serious problems in a million drinkers a year in Britain.[8] And it was associated with, among other things, 500,000 admissions to hospital, 14,000 psychiatric admissions, 65% of serious head injuries, 50% of murders, 40% of road accidents, one in three divorces, and one in three cases of child abuse. As these figures dramatically illustrate, alcohol causes many psychological, and physical, and social problems (see Box 7).

BOX 7	**Symptoms of problem drinking**
	Dependence Psychological problems • anxiety • depression • suicidal thinking Physical problems with damage to: • heart and blood vessels

- liver
- hormones and sexual function
- digestive system
- brain and nerves

Social problems

- debt
- marital problems
- children grow up with higher risk of problem drinking

Daniel's story is a more personal illustration of the problems alcohol can cause:

When Daniel was 10 his father died. He wasn't close to his mother and didn't respect her. Without the only figure of authority in his life he stopped caring about behaving himself. He got into fights at school, played truant, and started smoking.

By his early teens Daniel was a practised burglar, breaking into people's homes while they were out at work and he was meant to be at school. He stole video recorders and compact disc players and sold them to market traders.

Daniel began to drink with friends when he was 12. They got the alcohol from an older friend who looked 18. When he started going out with girls he was possessive, wondering if they would desert him like his father did. All too often, his possessiveness made the girls drop him. Daniel coped with the regular rejections by getting drunk.

At 20 Daniel was out of work. But he did have a steady girlfriend. When she got pregnant he was pleased, and he started planning family life together. She left him, though, and had an abortion. By this time Daniel had found that a constant level of alcohol in his body helped him to keep sadness, anxiety, and frustration at bay. He spent more than £20 a day on alcohol, paid for out of social security benefits, selling stolen goods, and borrowings from friends and his mother. The first drink in the morning made his persistent stomach ache worse but was worth having because it calmed his nerves and stopped his shakes. And besides, his only friends now were his drinking companions.

Soon after his girlfriend left, Daniel went on a drinking binge and got arrested for assaulting a security guard in the shopping precinct while drunk. When he came to court he was also found guilty of burglary. On the advice of a probation officer and a psychiatrist the court ordered Daniel to live in a probation hostel away from his home town, to accept outpatient treatment for his drinking problem, and to pay regular instalments of compensation to the security guard. If he didn't comply with this sentence over the next six months he would go to prison.

Dependence on alcohol, which Daniel had, has both psychological and physical components.

Alcohol Dependence

This is more or less the same as alcoholism, a word that professionals avoid these days because it is vague and stigmatizing. Most problem drinkers are not dependent. But those that are have particularly serious problems and need professional help. The key features of alcohol dependence are shown in Box 8.

BOX 8 **Key features of alcohol dependence**

The compulsion to drink alcohol is strong

Getting alcohol is more important than other daily activities

Coping with increasing doses of alcohol gets easier (tolerance develops)

Range of situations in which drinking occurs gets narrower

Repeated withdrawal symptoms are relieved by further drinking

Dependence rapidly resumes after a period of abstinence

Psychological Problems

Anxiety and depression are common among heavy drinkers. Some may have had these problems first, using drinking as a way of coping with unpleasant emotions. Personality disorders are also fairly common among drinkers. Around 15% of people with severe alcohol problems eventually die by suicide, some because of long-term depression, others on impulse when drunk.

Other alcohol-related problems that may need psychiatric help, like delirium tremens and long-term dementia, are clearly caused by brain damage. They are discussed later.

Physical Problems

Alcohol can damage many parts of the body including the heart, stomach, liver, and brain.

HEART AND BLOOD VESSELS

Alcohol is one of the commonest causes of high blood pressure, even at relatively low levels of intake: the risk among men starts to rise when weekly intake exceeds 14 units. High blood pressure, in turn, leads to heart attacks and strokes. A stroke happens when one of the main blood vessels supplying the brain becomes blocked by a blood clot or bleeds. Either event interrupts the blood supply and deprives that part of the brain of oxygen, killing some of the cells. Alcohol also impairs blood clotting, so increases the incidence of strokes in two ways.

The heart is particularly sensitive to alcohol's toxic effects. A single heavy binge can make the heart beat irregularly, causing palpitations. And drinking half a bottle of whisky or seven pints of beer a day for several months can seriously damage the heart muscle. The resulting condition, called cardiomyopathy, causes breathlessness and decreased stamina and sometimes sudden death. Many heavy drinkers have early signs of this damage which can be shown up by ultrasound tests.

LIVER
The liver is often damaged by alcohol, and cirrhosis of the liver is probably heavy drinking's best known physical consequence. Cirrhosis is the result of long-term inflammation of liver cells that have been exposed to high concentrations of alcohol. It causes irreversible scarring throughout the liver which impairs the organ's vital ability to break down toxic waste in the body. Symptoms of cirrhosis include jaundice, oedema (swelling of the soft tissues), hormone imbalances, and vomiting of blood. The build up of waste in the body can lead to brain damage.

Most drinkers do not develop cirrhosis. Many, however, have milder reversible forms of liver inflammation which make the organ's enzymes (the chemicals that regulate the liver's waste-removing functions) go haywire. Raised concentrations of these enzymes enter the blood and are detectable using simple blood tests. Knowing that there are early signs of liver damage can be a useful deterrent to heavy drinking, particularly given that the enzyme levels return to normal within a few weeks of stopping alcohol.

HORMONES AND SEXUAL FUNCTIONS
Even moderate drinking of around 25 units week can lower men's sperm counts, making them infertile. Sperm production recovers rapidly, within a few days, if alcohol is stopped.

Long-term heavy drinking can disrupt the body's hormone systems which regulate the menstrual cycle in women and sexual behaviour in both sexes. These changes can decrease sexual interest and energy and in the long run can make the ovaries and testicles shrink.

Sexual function may also be affected if a hormone problem called pseudo-Cushing's syndrome develops. This happens when alcohol damages the adrenal glands, producing the familiar picture of an overweight, round-faced and puffy-eyed drinker. Women with this syndrome tend to have irregular periods and excess facial hair; men become impotent. The syndrome can be cured by stopping alcohol.

DIGESTIVE SYSTEM

Alcohol can irritate the stomach and bowel causing gastritis, an inflammation of the stomach lining that causes persistent indigestion, peptic ulcers, diarrhoea, and even cancer of the pancreas and throat.

Heavy drinking can cause obesity and can stop people getting a normal diet. It contains many calories but few nutrients, and tends to reduce appetite. It also reduces the absorption from the stomach of B vitamins, which are essential for the healthy functioning of the brain and nerves.

BRAIN AND NERVES

Alcohol's commonest effect on the brain is intoxication. This means that it depresses the brain's normal functions, slowing down reaction times and reducing mental and physical control. Alcohol also reduces self-control and inhibitions, so that the mood someone was in before drinking – whether cheerful or miserable – is exaggerated. This explains why people get merry, tearful, or angry when drunk. Severe intoxication can lead to temporary loss of memory and even unconsciousness, which can be very dangerous if vomiting occurs.

Heavy drinking over many years can damage the nerves and brain by direct toxicity and by vitamin B deficiency. This deficiency may damage the nerves of the legs and feet in particular, causing a collection of abnormal sensations called peripheral neuropathy. The numbness may not be noticed until it is found by a doctor who tickles and pricks the feet and legs as part of a routine neurological examination. But some people suffer intense burning and tingling sensations and even unstable walking because the normal sense of where the feet are during movement is lost. Vitamin B deficiency from excessive drinking also causes a specific kind of brain damage called Wernicke's encephalopathy.

Wernicke's encephalopathy is a brain disease which develops suddenly, often when a big binge is superimposed on regular heavy drinking. Sufferers see double, lose their balance, and become very confused. Urgent treatment in hospital, giving vitamin B via a drip along with drying out, is nearly always necessary. Even with treatment this disease may progress to permanent brain damage and a dementia-like condition with loss of memory, loss of learning ability, and the need for full-time residential care. This permanent problem is called Korsakoff's syndrome after the Russian doctor who first described it. Bert, whose story follows, developed Korsakoff's syndrome:

Bert was 49. He had been dependent on alcohol since his 20s and had been homeless for many years. During his regular bouts of drinking he would eat no food, surviving on calories from alcohol alone.

After his latest bout of drinking Bert was found collapsed in a park and was taken to hospital for urgent treatment. He came round in a few hours and his double vision went after a couple of days. But Bert didn't know where he was, despite the nurses constant reminders, and he kept falling over.

Two weeks later Bert was much stronger but he still couldn't remember any of the nurses' names or find the ward bathroom. After a month he was still getting lost round the ward. He couldn't remember whether he had washed or eaten that day.

When the occupational therapist took Bert to the shops he forgot where they were going before even before reaching the hospital gates. He would walk out of the ward's occupational therapy kitchen and forget that he had left the gas cooker on. Clearly, Bert was unable to look after himself.

Despite all his disabilities Bert retained a rich store of old memories of his life before the brain damage and entertained other patients with his stories of life on the road. Eventually, a place was found for Bert in a staffed hostel where he could be cared for indefinitely.

Many patients with Korsakoff's syndrome languish in psychiatric wards for years, or end up in old people's homes despite being 20 or 30 years younger than the other residents. Bert was relatively lucky to be found a hostel, an environment that he knew well and liked because he had been homeless so long.

Two other kinds of brain damage result from heavy drinking. One is a mental illness similar to schizophrenia, with hallucinations and delusions. The other is due to generalized shrinkage of brain cells which causes a kind of dementia (see Chapter 4 for details on dementia) and sometimes results in damage to the cerebellum. The cerebellum is the part of the brain that controls and integrates movement. Drinkers with cerebellar damage look drunk even when sober because they walk very unsteadily and have a severe tremor when they move their hands.

Finally, the brain can go temporarily haywire causing delirium tremens or the DTs if someone who is dependent on alcohol suddenly stops drinking. Symptoms of the DTs include restlessness, anxiety, insomnia, confusion, hallucinations (classically of faces or spiders), and fits.

Social Problems

Many drinkers spend much more money than they can afford on alcohol. A number get into serious debt, often by getting loans from relatives and friends under false pretences.

Much of the burden of heavy drinking falls on users' families, who may have to cope with daily drunkenness and violence as well as financial problems. Alcohol ruins many marriages and is thought to be a factor in a third of divorces.

Children are particularly affected. Many child abusers are violent when drunk. And around a quarter of the offspring of alcohol-dependent parents grow up with alcohol problems themselves. Although some of this may be genetic, children seem to be most at risk when the whole family becomes demoralized and fragmented; if the family sticks together and somehow maintains a kind of harmony these children can actually end up as emotionally strong adults.[9] This need to stick together is just one of several good reasons why families of problem drinkers find the support of groups like AlAnon so helpful (see Appendix 2).

Treatments for Alcohol Problems
There are many different forms of treatment for problem drinking. This is partly because the range of problems is wide, because no single treatment has been shown to be much better than others, and partly because the professionals who provide treatment have differing attitudes and backgrounds. One broad distinction among treatments is their location – outpatient services are mainly for people with less severe problems while hospital wards are mainly for those with emergencies and more severe long-term problems.

Outpatient Treatment
Outpatient treatment is ideal for drinkers who are not dependent on alcohol or are only mildly so and are able to get on with most aspects of daily life. The aim of treatment is usually to control drinking at a lower and less problematic level. Using drinking diaries (see p. 167) patients are helped to understand their patterns of drinking, along with the related social and emotional factors. Strategies to reduce drinking can then be devised.

For someone whose heavy drinking usually occurs in pubs, perhaps resulting in drink-driving convictions and marital problems, the strategy might include avoiding rounds, stretching drinks by sipping not gulping, putting the glass down between sips, going to the pub nearer closing time, and alternating drinks with low-alcohol or alcohol-free beer.

Drinking to avoid unhappiness can be helped by counselling and practical advice. For instance a married woman who drinks heavily when alone in the evenings might be helped to negotiate with her husband for more support. Perhaps he could come home at a more reasonable time on certain days; either to be with her or to babysit while she goes to an evening class.

Treatment in Hospital

Intensive treatment in hospital is usually reserved for emergencies, when outpatient treatment fails, and for people with severe problems and dependency. It is almost impossible for people who are severely dependent on alcohol to cut down their intake without being dried out: they might get the DTs (see p. 179) without proper treatment and supervision.

Drying out (detoxification) involves stopping alcohol completely and taking decreasing doses of other drugs, usually tranquillizers, for a week or so to control the withdrawal symptoms. This is usually done in a ward. But patients can live at home and come in daily for treatment or even receive treatment at home from community nurses, as long as there are other people at home to keep an eye on them.

After drying out there are several options for treatment. The following stories explain what may happen:

Jim was 70. He had been a member of Alcoholics Anonymous (AA) for 20 years and had stayed dry nearly all that time. But in late retirement, when Jim had time on his hands and failing physical health, he started drinking heavily again. After being dried out in hospital Jim stayed there for daily group therapy over four weeks. He went along to AA meetings from the hospital and when he was discharged he re-established his old network of support through AA. Jim saw his GP for regular checks but did not have to go to hospital again.

Bob was discharged from hospital after drying out, taking disulfiram (trade name Antabuse) to deter him from drinking again. If he drank, the alcohol and Antabuse would react with each other, making him vomit and feel ill. During the three months of treatment with the drug Bob knew he would not succumb to the temptation to drink and returned to work. He also attended a weekly outpatient group that taught him how to deal with difficult situations without drinking. The group leader set Bob and the other members homework tasks, for instance making a point of going swimming on the way home from work on Fridays instead of going to the pub.

Frank had been thrown out by his wife. He had nowhere to live when discharged from hospital after drying out, so he went to a 'dry hostel' where he was not allowed to drink. He attended the clinic every day for support and encouragement. After a month his social worker found him a place in a smaller dry house with a therapeutic programme. This meant regular residents' meetings, communal cooking and household chores, and one-to-one counselling. Six months later Frank was ready to live in a bedsit in a nearby town, from where he went for counselling sessions at a local advice centre.

Margaret was already involved with the social services before treatment because she had got so drunk at home one day that her small daughter, Hannah, had wandered off into a busy street. After drying out, Margaret and her boyfriend attended a family support centre which helped them to cope better with Hannah. Margaret also spent one day a week at the alcohol clinic, having treatment for her anxiety.

Alcoholics Anonymous
As the name implies AA is exclusively for sufferers and ex-sufferers from alcohol problems who hold meetings which people attend without giving their names. The organization also offers individual support, in person or on the phone, from experienced AA members. Meetings are held regularly

in most towns and contact numbers are listed in phone books, directories of local services and local papers.

Meetings have an inspirational theme, rather like evangelical and 'born again' religious gatherings. Indeed, AA's basic philosophy or creed, which originated in the US, is belief in a higher power from whom drinkers can draw strength. The power need not be God, however, and members do not have to be religious or churchgoers. The other main strand of AA's philosophy is that the best person to understand an alcoholic is another alcoholic. During AA meetings members talk about the effects of alcohol on their lives, and how following AA's philosophy enabled them to return to sobriety.

Alcoholics Anonymous presents one clear view of alcohol problems; namely that sufferers have a progressive disease caused by a kind of allergy to alcohol over which they have no control. Members believe firmly in total and life-long abstinence: the aim is always to be sober today, rather than for the next six months or in ten years.

The only requirement for AA membership is the desire to stop drinking. Abstinence is achieved through mutual support, the acceptance of AA's philosophy, and certain practical ways to alter lifestyle and daily routines. Practical points are reinforced with simple slogans like 'one day at a time', 'one drink equals one drunk' and 'I am responsible'.

Some people with alcohol problems find AA hard to take. But the organization has more than 1.5 million members in nearly 100 countries worldwide. And two spin-offs from AA do a lot to advise and support families of drinkers: Al-Anon is for spouses and partners, Al-Ateen is for children.

Two further voluntary organizations provide support and information on alcohol problems: Alcohol Concern and Accept. The national addresses of all these groups are given in Appendix 2.

Outcome of Treatment

No one really agrees on what constitutes successful treatment for alcohol problems. Some experts believe the aim should be controlled drinking, others that abstinence is the key. Still others regard solving social and family problems as the most important aim. And, of course, what matters most to drinkers may be different again. Still, a few points about treatment are worth noting.

It may be obvious, but research now shows that younger people with only moderate problems are better off with controlled drinking. Those who are over 40 and have long-lasting and severe problems, particularly dependence, are safer with abstinence.

There is some evidence that GPs and doctors on general medical wards can reduce patients' moderately heavy drinking for up to a year, with just one session of brief advice on cutting down. A study of 100 men with severe alcohol problems showed that such simple advice was as successful as intensive treatment that included drug therapy, counselling for patients and their wives, and AA meetings.[10]

Alcoholics Anonymous says that around 45% of members at a typical meeting have been sober for 2–10 years. It is impossible to verify this because the organization's anonymity rules out keeping any records. But it does suggest that people who feel comfortable with AA's approach stand a good chance of staying dry.

PROBLEM DRUGS OTHER THAN ALCOHOL

Other mind-altering drugs cause a range of general problems – physical, psychological, social and economic, and legal. But certain drugs (see Box 9) cause specific problems related to their different properties and modes of use. They are detailed below.

The last three groups of drugs are legally available to adults in Britain. Solvents and nicotine are sold over the counter in every high street; tranquillizers are prescribed by doctors. But all three types of drug cause considerable problems.

BOX 9 | **Problem drugs other than alcohol**
- Opiates
- Dance drugs
- Other stimulants
- Hallucinogens
- Cannabis
- Solvents
- Tranquillizers
- Nicotine

Groups of Problem Drugs

Opiates
Opiates are drugs made from opium, which comes from the sap of poppy seed pods. The most common street opiates are heroin, morphine, pethidine, and codeine. Heroin is usually manufactured illegally; the others are obtained through burglaries on chemists shops and through illegal import.

Opiates may be smoked, eaten, or injected. They produce a feeling of euphoria, a 'high,' and a pleasant carefree state of mind with a sense of detachment from mundane reality. Users quickly tolerate and need increasingly large doses and dependence develops rapidly.

Severe withdrawal symptoms start within hours of using up the supply. They are like a bad dose of flu, with aches and pains, runny nose, diarrhoea, cramps, restlessness, irritability, and strong craving for the drug.

Some people manage to live relatively normal lives, taking enough opiates to ward off withdrawal symptoms but not enough to cause a constant high. The greatest harm comes from three things: infection through dirty needles (see p. 193), overdose (which reduces the breathing rate and can lead to coma or death), and crime.

Treatment for opiate dependence, like that for alcohol

dependence, starts with drying out – usually over a long period of time and through an outpatient clinic or health centre. Methadone is prescribed as a substitute for the illegal opiate. It is longer-acting than heroin and therefore causes more gradual withdrawal; it can be taken by mouth, and it does not produce psychologically addictive highs like heroin. Getting regular prescriptions of methadone also releases users from the need to raise money through crime. This combined approach is called, reasonably enough, harm reduction.

Subsequent treatment is much like that for alcohol problems. Outcome of treatment for opiate dependence is not always encouraging. In a study in London four-fifths of users achieved abstinence during inpatient drying out, but only 17% of those treated as outpatients completed treatment and stopped their drugs.[11] Yet most users are treated as outpatients; inpatient facilities are few and far between and it is difficult to persuade users to agree to admission. Those that are treated out of hospital often continue to use their illegal drugs as well, and some sell the methadone.

Dance Drugs

The early 1990s has seen the rapid rise of rave culture among young people in Britain. A rave is a huge organized party, usually lasting all night, at which partygoers dance continuously to music that is often mixed on the spot. Raves are advertised through word of mouth, underground magazines, and pirate radio stations, and hundreds of teenagers attend for around £10–20 a head. At first ravers did not tend to drink alcohol, instead they had cold soft drinks and ice creams to cool themselves down. Ravers get hot for two reasons – dancing non-stop and taking stimulant drugs.

The stimulants used at raves and at some night clubs include drugs that have been around for years like amphetamines, cocaine, and poppers (amyl nitrite). Ravers also use well-known hallucinogenic drugs like LSD (lysergic acid) and angel dust (phencyclidine or PCP).

But rave culture has its own, newer, drugs including ecstasy (an amphetamine derivative with street names including E, XTC, and Dennis the Menace, and the chemical name methylenedioxymethamphetamine, or MDMA for short) and ketamine (a hallucinogenic drug, street name K). Ecstasy is manufactured illegally, mainly in continental Europe. It is taken by mouth as tablets and capsules. It is a stimulant and a partial hallucinogen. It induces a 'rush', a feeling of energy, euphoria, and alertness, in which there may be heightened sensations and occasionally hallucinations. This is followed later by relaxation and calm. Ecstasy's risks include psychological dependence; overstimulation with insomnia, anxiety and later depression; and, very occasionally, sudden death. In Britain since 1988 around 15 deaths have resulted from ecstasy. These have occurred when the stimulant effects of ecstasy, combined with dancing in a hot place and losing too much fluid through sweating, have caused severe overheating with raised blood pressure and pulse rate.

Ketamine is a drug used medically as an injection to start general anaesthesia. It was first used illegally in 1991–2 as an extra ingredient of ecstasy tablets and capsules and is now used separately.[12] Ketamine depresses brain activity; hence its ability to anaesthetize people. Users say it produces a state of profound unreality. They feel as if they have left their bodies and the real world because the drug inhibits movement and reduces real sensations to almost nothing, while causing hallucinations. Some users say this state, which lasts about half an hour, is like a near-death experience. Indeed, some feel completely indifferent to whether they are alive or dead, a feeling that could be dangerous in the crowds at large raves. Not much is known about long-term use, although some users report having 'flashbacks' or re-experienced hallucinations after the drug's other effects have worn off. In theory, ketamine could cause memory problems. A few cases of dependence on injected ketamine have occurred.

Other Stimulants
This group of drugs includes amphetamines and cocaine. Amphetamine (speed or whizz) is mainly synthesized illegally. Other drugs in the same group (trade name Tenuate

Dospan and Apisate) are prescribed drugs used in slimming clinics to suppress appetite: they are sold on the black market. Cocaine was once a widely used medical drug because it is a local anaesthetic, and many drugs related to it are still used in this way. It was also the ingredient that once gave Coca Cola its name (although it is no longer present in cola drinks). Now cocaine and its street derivatives, including crack, are almost entirely made illegally.

All these drugs can be eaten, smoked, sniffed, or injected. They increase alertness and energy and make users feel exhilarated, powerful, and sometimes aggressive. They prevent sleep and reduce appetite.

Although stimulants do not cause physical withdrawal syndromes, users may become psychologically dependent on them. Long-term and even short-term use of stimulants in high doses carry the risk of heart problems and, occasionally, sudden death. Amphetamines can also cause a psychotic illness like acute schizophrenia, lasting days or weeks. Cocaine withdrawal can cause depression that is so sudden and severe that users call it 'crash'. Antidepressant drugs can sometimes relieve this depressed state.

Hallucinogens

Ecstasy and ketamine – partial hallucinogens – have been described already. The main drug in this group is lysergic acid diethylamide (LSD) which is made and distributed illegally in several oral forms including tablets, capsules, and impregnated squares of paper printed with graphic symbols ('magic' mushrooms contain similar drugs). LSD causes 'trips' away from reality, with altered thinking and sensation that includes exaggerated perception of colours and sounds. Complicated hallucinations may occur and, depending on the user's mood, these can be pleasant and beautiful or frightening and threatening. Trips last up to 12 hours and can, not surprisingly, be disruptive and even dangerous. Users may act on their hallucinations, perhaps by wandering out into the street or trying to drive, and get into accidents.

Long-term use of LSD is not medically dangerous, although

the occurrence of flashbacks (see ketamine) may be due to some kind of transient brain damage. Physical dependence does not occur.

Cannabis

Cannabis is the most widely used illegal drug in Britain. Around 7% of the population uses it.[13] It has many street names including dope, marijuana, pot, hash, grass, ganga and blow. It is available on the black market in resin, oil, and herb forms, all of which can be smoked. Herbal and resin forms are usually smoked with tobacco.

Drugs related to cannabis are used to treat nausea in patients receiving cancer chemotherapy. And some researchers say that cannabis should be licensed for medicinal use as a pain killer.

Like alcohol, cannabis makes users feel relaxed, happy and talkative as long as they start off in a good mood. Some people say it is an aphrodisiac, though this probably just reflects a general lifting of inhibitions. Cannabis heightens awareness of sound and colour but reduces concentration.

High doses of cannabis can make users confused and transiently psychotic and paranoid. There is some debate among psychiatrists whether prolonged and regular use of cannabis can cause a long-term psychotic illness like schizophrenia. The latest consensus is that it does not, but that it seems to increase the risk of developing schizophrenia by two or three times.[14] This has been suggested as one reason why schizophrenia is diagnosed most frequently among Afro-Caribbean men, who tend to use cannabis regularly.

The other long-term health risks – bronchitis and lung cancer – are caused by the tars and other products of cannabis smoke. Cannabis has no other specific risks to health but users face one big problem, namely crime and prosecution. Some experts say cannabis should be legalized like nicotine and alcohol, relieving the crime problem associated with its use.

Solvents

This group of chemicals includes butane fuel for cigarette lighters, acetone nail varnish, some aerosols, and glues containing toluene or acetone. When their volatile fumes are inhaled, usually from a plastic bag held up to the face, they produce intoxication rather like that caused by alcohol. A telltale rash may develop round the mouth and nose, caused by the irritating fumes.

Solvents are used as drugs mainly by young teenagers, particularly boys. A survey of 25,000 children in Britain in 1987 showed that one in eight of 14–15-year-olds had used solvents.[15]

High doses of solvents can cause hallucinations and severe intoxication which leads to coma or even death. Most of the 150 or so deaths a year, however, result from inhalation of vomit by unconscious users. Long-term use of solvents containing toluene can damage the part of the brain that coordinates movement, the cerebellum.[16] This leads to a drunken-looking and unsteady walk, shaking of the hands, and problems with eye movements. Mild degrees of cerebellar damage will resolve if the solvent is stopped.

No one knows for sure whether solvent use can dull the intellect. Heavy use is commonest among boys with already chaotic behaviour, truancy, and poor educational performance, and it is difficult to unravel these pre-existing problems from any that might arise after use. Solvents do not cause physical dependence.

There is no specific treatment for users. For most of them solvent use is a passing phase; most stop using the drugs spontaneously by school leaving age, perhaps because use is mainly a group activity. For the few with persistent problems counselling, family therapy and social support may help.

Tranquillizers

In 1991 government figures showed that around 19 million prescriptions for benzodiazepine tranquillizers and sleeping tablets were issued by GPs in Britain. This group includes diazepam (trade name Valium), temazepam (Normison), nitrazepam (Mogadon) and lorazepam (Ativan).

The extent of dependence problems associated with these drugs is discussed in Chapter 1. Benzodiazepines are strongly addictive. Withdrawal symptoms include severe anxiety, insomnia, nausea, diarrhoea, and sometimes confusion and convulsions. Coming off benzodiazepines should be done very gradually to avoid these symptoms. If drying out in hospital is necessary it can be done over as little as a week or two using other, less addictive drugs in the same group.

As well as the problems among people who are prescribed benzodiazepines there is also considerable illegal use of these drugs, particularly in Scotland. Prescribed benzodiazepines enter the black market when people trade them for street drugs. Some illegal users crush the tablets or open up the capsules to make injectable forms of benzodiazepine.

Nicotine
Around 100,000 deaths a year are attributed to smoking tobacco. Most smokers smoke regularly because they are psychologically dependent on the drug nicotine, which is the active ingredient of tobacco. Nicotine calms the nerves, or at least clears the brain. But it also stimulates the release of the hormone adrenaline into the blood, which gives smokers a mild 'buzz'.

The message about smoking's risks is getting through to most adult smokers now, and many manage to give up spontaneously. Help for smokers who cannot give up on their own includes counselling, group therapy, hypnosis, and acupuncture – all of which work for some people. Replacement therapy using nicotine chewing gum or nicotine patches (sticking plasters impregnated with the drug) reduces craving and has few side effects, none of them serious. Both forms of prescribed nicotine therapy result in between one-fifth and one-quarter of heavy smokers abstaining completely during follow-up periods of several months.[17]

Problems Related to Ways that Drugs are Procured and Used

Drugs and Crime

The relationship between drugs and crime has three strands. Firstly, many drug users raise money through crime to buy their drugs. Secondly, the manufacture, import, and distribution of illegal drug depends on networks of organized crime, both nationally and internationally. Thirdly, British law includes a range of drugs offences, not all of which are limited to manufacturers and distributors. Drug users also break the law.

The Misuse of Drugs Act 1971 outlaws the manufacture, possession and supply of certain controlled drugs. The Act puts drugs into three groups – classes A, B, and C – in order of dangerousness and enforceable penalties.

Class A includes opium, heroin, methadone, morphine, pethidine, cocaine, crack, lysergic acid (LSD), ecstasy, phencyclidine, and processed magic mushrooms, plus any class-B substance prepared for injection. Possession gets up to seven years in jail, trafficking can attract a life sentence.

Class B includes amphetamines, barbiturates, cannabis, cannabis resin, codeine, and dihydrocodeine (DF118). Class C drugs include benzodiazepine tranquillizers like diazepam (Valium), and mild amphetamine-like drugs. If class-C tranquillizers are in the form of prescribable medicines it is not an offence to possess them, even if they have not been prescribed. But it is illegal to sell them.

Infections Related to Drug Injection: HIV and Hepatitis B

People who inject illegal drugs are the fastest growing group of AIDS sufferers in Europe, and in some parts of the Continent they account for half of all newly diagnosed cases, according to the World Health Organization. In 1986 there were around 75,000–150,000 people in Britain taking heroin and other opiates, half of whom were injecting, and about the same number were injecting amphetamine.[18]

The virus that causes AIDS is called the human immunodeficiency virus, HIV for short. Like another virus which causes liver disease, hepatitis B virus, it is transmitted through blood, by unsterile needles, and through sex. There is an effective vaccine against hepatitis B virus, and the problems it causes – liver inflammation, jaundice, nausea and abdominal pain – usually clear up eventually. But HIV infection cannot yet be prevented by vaccination or cured and AIDS – the final stage of the illness with cancers and severe infection – is always fatal.

Drug users catch these infections in two ways: by unsafe sex without condoms and by sharing needles and syringes, or 'works', that have not been sterilized. Ideally drug users should not inject drugs. But, when they do, they should use new sterilized needles and syringes available from doctors and chemists and should throw them away safely after use. At the very least, users can clean their injecting equipment by soaking it in strong bleach; but this does not guarantee absolute safety from infection. Some users get more out of injecting themselves if they share the emotional experience with other drug users; and sometimes this means sharing needles. But this is just not worth the risk. (Incidentally, dirty needles can transmit other infections, particularly bacterial ones that cause septicaemia, or blood poisoning. This is treatable with antibiotics but may be bad enough to warrant admission to hospital.)

Safe sex often goes by the board among drug users. This is partly because many drugs, including alcohol, reduce inhibitions and increase desire while impairing concentration and consciousness and awareness of what is happening. And some drug users, particularly those using expensive 'hard' drugs, earn money through prostitution. Inevitably, this often involves unsafe sex.

Services for drug users spend a lot of energy and time trying to reduce the risks of infections. In some areas clinics and general practice health centres run successful needle exchange schemes, providing free sterile syringes and needles and disposing safely of used equipment.

Self-Help and Family Support for People with Drug Problems

Many local and national voluntary organizations offer advice, support and help to users and their families. National agencies include Narcotics Anonymous, Turning Point, and Release, whose addresses are given in Appendix 2.

Parents of users sometimes need a lot of information and support. As one drugs researcher, Dr Russell Newcombe, said in a Sunday newspaper, parents think that a couple of joints is the path to Armageddon:

> If you consider how many people use drugs, and how many have not been harmed, it is clear that responsible drug taking need not be the worst horror imaginable. Nor does there seem any likelihood that the young will stop using drugs ... All the evidence shows that parents going berserk does not work. Understanding what is going on and being vigilant is the best protection parents can offer.[19]

6 EATING DISORDERS

Are We What We Eat?

> Subdue your appetites, my dears, and you've con-
> quered human nature.
> From *Nicholas Nickleby* by Charles Dickens

Few of us sit down to a meal determined purely by our stomachs: our minds make demands too. Looking at recipe books stimulates the appetite even if the body is not really hungry, and eating just before going to a supermarket lessens the likelihood of filling the trolley with unaffordable titbits. Certain religions and cultures have special codes for preparing and eating food. But even those of us who think our eating is quite spontaneous are affected by social pressures, particularly in our families. Most families get together only at meal times and, if the pattern of regular communal meals breaks down, it is surprisingly easy for close relatives to go for days without speaking more than a few words to each other.

A meal can mean much more than its face value. Even a quick snack can be a labour of love for the cook, usually the mother, who will probably feel hurt if it is refused. Emotions are not only aroused by issues around eating, they can also affect eating patterns in the first place. Unhappiness usually reduces appetite (perhaps this is why unhappy people say they feel fed up), but can also lead to overeating and using food as a comforting reward. Perhaps this is a throwback to infancy when babies depend on their mouths for pleasure and security as well as for feeding.

Sigmund Freud said that adults could become abnormally

interested in (or fixated on) oral pleasures like eating and smoking if problems in infancy prevented them from growing out of thinking that their mouths were all-important. Other psychologists have suggested similar theories linking food with pleasure and sex. Even sceptics cannot deny that a romantic dinner is an effective seduction device. Advertisers of food understand this: cream cakes are naughty but nice, chocolates are delivered by mysteriously ravishing intruders, and instant coffee guarantees everlasting love.

In some ways, therefore, society emphasizes the pleasures of food. But in present-day Western societies the most indulgent and enjoyable foods have acquired a mostly negative image. This is partly because of widespread medical advice to cut down on fattening foods, to exercise, and to stay lean. This general message is important and is justified by the scientific facts, although some advice may have been overdone – for instance, recent studies suggest that only people with inherited tendencies to high blood cholesterol need to drastically reduce cholesterol in their diets. Anyway, most people in the West now believe that being overweight is unhealthy. Many also think that it is unattractive, sometimes to the point of making big people completely unsexy or even socially unacceptable. These social influences, reinforced by fashion and by role models in the media and arts, affect eating patterns and body image.

Interestingly, these pressures do not seem to make the majority of society lose weight. In Britain, France, the US and most other Western countries men and women are getting bigger. The British government says that in 1986–7 one in twelve men and one in eight women were obese. Clothes retailers report that average bust, waist and hip measurements have increased in recent years. This partly reflects mankind's general tendency to get taller and bigger as people are better fed and less stunted by disease. Among women it may also reflect widespread use of the oral contraceptive pill, which can cause weight increase and breast enlargement.

Although social pressure to be thin does not seem to make modern men and women lose weight, it makes them want to.

Dieting is endemic. The dieter's organization Weightwatchers now has some 150,000 members in Britain alone. Women in particular are subjected to the pressure to lose weight. Yet women rather than men also have good reasons to find dieting hard: these include the pill, pregnancy, and much greater involvement than men in preparing and serving food. It is no wonder that the problems that doctors call eating disorders – anorexia and bulimia nervosa, compulsive eating – occur much more commonly among women than men.

ANOREXIA NERVOSA

> One can never be too rich. One can never be too thin.
> *Duchess of Windsor (Wallis Simpson)*[1]

Anorexia is a medical term meaning loss of appetite, and it is a symptom of many physical illnesses. Patients in hospital with physical problems may hear doctors use the term as they stand round the bed, and wrongly assume that a psychiatrist will be called. Anorexia nervosa, however, is a well-defined serious illness which may not involve loss of appetite even though the anorexic (or anorectic) sufferer barely eats. Many people assume that it is a modern illness, prompted by the fashions for slimming and for women to be boyishly thin, but it was first described, named, and recognized as a psychological problem 120 years ago. Then the recommended treatment was firm supervision of food intake so that sufferers could no longer starve themselves, combined with counselling for their families. Little has changed since then.

Anorexia nervosa usually starts in adolescence and young adulthood. But it can occur at any age, even in elderly people. It is about 10 times more common among women than men. It affects about 1–2% of teenagers and college students and there are about 120,000 sufferers in Britain at any time.

Symptoms of Anorexia Nervosa
Anorexia nervosa involves a wide range of physical and psychological problems, which are summarized in Box 1.

BOX 1

> ## Symptoms of anorexia nervosa
>
> *Physical symptoms*
> - Loss of at least one-quarter of normal weight
> - Starvation
> - Loss of periods
>
> *Psychological symptoms*
> - Fear of normal weight
> - Distortion of body image
>
> People with anorexia nervosa may speed up weight loss from dieting by vomiting, purging and excessively exercising

Physical Symptoms
The primary physical problem in anorexia nervosa is severe weight loss, usually of at least one-quarter of the normal weight for the person's build. For example, a woman of medium frame and height of 5ft 4in (163 cm) should weigh between 8½ and 9½ stones (56–62 kg) and a loss of one-quarter would be about 3 stones (19 kg), taking her down to about six (38 kg).

The weight loss is caused by self-starvation. The physical effects of starvation include feeling cold all the time (particularly in the hands and feet), tiredness and anaemia, fainting caused by low blood pressure and slow pulse, constipation, osteomalacia (thinning and weakening of the bones), swollen ankles, and hormone disturbances (affecting the menstrual cycle, thyroid function, and body growth). Fine downy hair called lanugo may grow on the face and body, perhaps in a biological attempt to keep warm. Coldness and the desire to hide the extent of weight loss also make sufferers wear layers of bulky clothes. Death from starvation takes a long time, but serious physical illness and even death from a heart attack can occur suddenly if the balance of water and minerals, particularly potassium, in the body is altered too much by self-starving.

Severe weight loss in women prevents periods. Menstruation usually starts in puberty, between the ages of 10 and 13, in response to a natural increase in weight over what scientists call the pubertal weight threshold – about four-fifths of final adult weight. If weight goes down below this threshold again the hormones which control the menstrual cycle go haywire and periods stop. The technical term for absence of periods is amenorrhoea and in anorexia nervosa it may be primary, for example when a teenager of 16 has never had a period, or secondary when someone who has had periods for some time stops having them. Evolution probably explains why adequate feeding switches on the hormones and organs that allow menstruation. Many animals do not ovulate until winter ends and adequate food is available. Human ovulation seems to depend on feeding in a similar way.

Psychological Symptoms

People with anorexia nervosa are often said to have a fear of fatness. In fact fear of normal weight and of looking like a normal adult is probably even more important. After all, many women and men are afraid of being fat these days, but that does not make them all anorectic. It does make many people diet, though, to reduce their weights till they reach certain targets. Some people with anorexia nervosa start dieting because they are initially overweight. But they keep dieting and do not stop when they reach normal weight. This is because they have distorted images of their own bodies, thinking they are still big when they have lost a considerable amount of weight. Researchers have asked sufferers to estimate their own waist and hip measurements and they have shown that people with anorexia nervosa grossly overestimate their size ('I wish I could lose my fat tummy' – Pat, 5 stone 3 pounds).

False perception of body image may actually increase as sufferers get more emaciated. This seems to involve a general inability to estimate size, even of inanimate objects and distances between them, and is thought to be the effect of starvation on the part of the brain that detects size. People with anorexia nervosa often seem oblivious to their physical deterioration too, strongly denying that anything is wrong. They say that they just don't feel like eating much, or that they are simply on a diet.

Sufferers do not, however, go off food. Complete fasting suppresses appetite after a day or two, but eating usually stimulates it again with a vengeance. Someone who eats small amounts irregularly may get very hungry. People with anorexia nervosa do not fast completely. Thus, they often have to resist good appetites and strong cravings. Many direct their obsession with food into an interest in cooking. Many take up catering as a career.

Strict calorie-controlled dieting is not usually enough to cause the severe weight loss seen in anorexia, often because other people expect and insist on proper eating. Many sufferers prevent adequate absorption of food by vomiting or taking laxatives. To dispel feelings of bloatedness after unavoidable meals some take diuretics ('water tablets') which are normally prescribed for high blood pressure or can be bought over the counter, in mild or homeopathic forms, to dispel premenstrual water retention. Many also take strenuous exercise, to an obsessive and excessive degree. Knowing that drastic weight-reducing behaviour is abnormal and likely to attract unwanted attention, sufferers often do these things secretly.

Jane's story sums up many of these points:

> Fifteen-year-old Jane seemed to be becoming a bit of a loner, having been a cheerful and gregarious child. She was obviously growing up quite quickly now: her periods had started some time ago, she was getting tall and losing her puppy fat. But normal growing up wasn't enough to explain her withdrawal from social life.

Perhaps she was worried about her GCSE exams; but she had always done well academically, and her teachers had no complaints. Whenever her mother tried to talk to her, Jane said she felt fine. Jane would disappear off to her room as soon as she got home from school and did not spend much time with the family. She had fallen out with her friends and her only interest was running, a favourite sport that seemed to consume her these days. Nothing traumatic had happened in the family recently, except the usual teenage rows: she had always got on fairly well with her brother Simon and her parents.

Jane's mother asked the family doctor for advice. He reassured her that it was probably just a passing phase. But the phase continued, and communication became so bad that Jane even refused to join the family for meals. She said that she had too much homework to do, and that she would just grab a sandwich. Once she had finished her work she would go out for a run – to train for the school team, she said. One night Jane's father saw her sitting at the side of the road as he was driving back from work. She was hunched forwards, head in hands, and panting. He stopped, and found her breathless and dizzy, and too weak even to argue when he put her into the car and drove her home. Jane denied feeling ill, but her parents noticed how thin and pale she was looking and insisted she went to the doctor the next day.

The story unravelled quickly at the doctor's. Examined without her layers of jumpers and baggy jeans, Jane was obviously very thin. She weighed a stone less than she had at the previous year's school medical. She was anaemic, but heavy periods were not to blame because she hadn't had any for months. The doctor urged Jane to stop dieting. She had been missing lunch at school by telling staff she had sandwiches, and eating only unfattening things at home.

For a while, things seemed to improve. Jane seemed

more cheerful and was eating normal meals again. But then her mother found her making herself sick after a meal. Nothing her parents tried seemed to get through to her. Watching her at mealtimes ended in arguments, and all attempts to talk things over were just shrugged off. Jane insisted that there was nothing wrong and that her parents were being stupid. After six months Jane was so thin that she looked seriously ill and was often taking days off school with colds and flu. Her doctor warned that the dieting was out of control, and that Jane now had anorexia nervosa. She weighed less than six stones. He offered to see Jane once a week, and said that he wanted to refer her to a psychiatrist at the local general hospital. She refused. The doctor and Jane's parents all felt they were treading a thin line between trying to help her and making things worse, and they agreed to stick it out for another few weeks.

One month later Jane was rushed to hospital after taking a handful of painkillers. She recovered from the overdose within a day or two but she was so thin and starved that she needed tube feeding and injections of vitamins. She agreed, reluctantly, to go to a psychiatric unit for young people.

Causes of Anorexia Nervosa

There is rarely one single reason why someone develops anorexia nervosa. Inheritance, mental and physical illnesses, and teenage emotional problems, as well as long-term family stresses and social pressures may all put someone at special risk of developing it. Stressful events, particularly in teenage, may then trigger the illness in vulnerable people (see Box 2).[2]

BOX 2	**Probable causes of anorexia nervosa**
	Risk factors
	● Family stresses
	● Social pressure

- Inheritance
- Mental and physical illnesses

Triggers
- Stressful life events

Risk Factors

INHERITANCE
Anorexia nervosa runs in families along with other problem behaviours such as overeating and addictions. Up to 10% of sisters of sufferers develop the illness, compared with 1–2% of the general population. This may be because members of the same family are brought up in the same environment, although it may mean that the tendency to be anorectic is inherited.

Studies show that 50% of identical twins of sufferers also develop anorexia nervosa compared with only 10% of non-identical twins. This suggests that inheritance is more important than upbringing in making people prone to this illness. Most professionals working with anorectics, however, feel that this proneness only leads to the full-blown illness if there are additional social and psychological pressures.

MENTAL AND PHYSICAL ILLNESSES
Problems like depression, anxiety and personality disorder (see Chapter 7) can all occur with anorexia nervosa. Depression can also cause weight loss that might be confused with anorexia nervosa, although rarely to below three-quarters of normal weight. Physical illnesses affecting menstruation or weight, or both, must also be ruled out before deciding on a diagnosis of anorexia nervosa. Hormone problems in the ovary and brain can interrupt periods. Diabetes, thyroid overactivity, bowel diseases, and other serious illnesses can cause weight loss. GPs can detect these problems, however, by physical examination and tests.

TEENAGE EMOTIONAL PROBLEMS

Refusal to eat is a powerful way to upset other people, particularly mothers. Meals are, perhaps, the most direct evidence of a mother's care; rejecting food is a sure way to cause havoc in the family. Self-starvation may also be a way of exercising some kind of power and control when teenagers feel generally powerless or out of control. It is too simplistic to say that a deliberately manipulative teenager says 'I'm getting too big, and I want to upset Mum, so I think I'll stop eating.' But anorectics who get better through therapy often come out with this kind of explanation themselves, even though they were not consciously aware of what was happening at the time.

Precipitating Factors or Triggers

Anorexia nervosa often starts soon after a stressful event. That the event actually causes the onset of illness is difficult to prove. Teenagers have to face taking exams, finding work or going to college, leaving home, having relationships, dealing with sex – all of which may just coincidentally precede the illness. But it makes sense that all these reminders of impending adulthood, combined with the physical changes of puberty, may be very scary. Perhaps losing weight and reversing these physical changes makes returning to the time before puberty seem a safe alternative to adulthood for some girls.

The role of acute stress is borne out by studies of people who develop anorexia nervosa in later life. These suggest that big life events, like those described on p. 10, trigger the onset.

Treatment for Anorexia Nervosa

Because of the gradual onset of the illness and the lack of an obvious single cause, it is quite unusual for sufferers to look for help spontaneously. Even confiding in friends may be hard, given that many people with anorexia nervosa seem to lose the ability to get close to anyone. Talking to a stranger who understands is often easier: the Eating Disorders Association, a self-help group, provides advice and support for both sufferers and their families (see Appendix 2 for address).

Once someone with anorexia nervosa does agree to professional help, the GP is the first port of call. GPs can confirm the diagnosis and rule out other illnesses, both physical and mental. They have three main options if sufferers from anorexia nervosa agree to be helped: treatment in the surgery or at home, referral to a psychiatrist, or referral to an internal medicine specialist (a physician, as opposed to a surgeon).

The choice will depend on the severity of the symptoms and, to some extent, on how much time and experience GPs have in treating anorexia nervosa.

Both psychiatrists and physicians will provide outpatient treatment, as long as sufferers are still coping adequately with daily life and are not too physically ill. The first hurdle they have to clear is the denial and resistance to interference that many sufferers have – they feel that there is nothing much wrong and that no one else understands. Doctors and therapists have to try particularly hard to get on well with sufferers. Treatment will not get very far without cooperation. The range of treatments is summarized in Box 3.

BOX 3

> **Treatments for anorexia nervosa**
>
> *Physical*
> - Refeeding
> - Drugs (occasionally)
>
> *Psychological*
> - Behaviour therapy
> - Counselling
> - Psychotherapy and family therapy

Doctors treating anorexia nervosa need a clear idea of the extent of the problem – not just the physical symptoms, but also the abnormal eating patterns. They may ask sufferers to keep diaries of everything eaten and of every attempt at weight loss such as vomiting, laxative use and strenuous exercise. As well as helping the helpers, these records bring home to sufferers just how abnormal things have become. Diaries are then used to set a framework for gaining weight. It is very important to aim for gradual weight gain (about 0.5–1 kg/1–2 lb per week) so that bodies and minds can adjust slowly without feeling overfed, scared, or out of control. A target weight must be agreed by the doctor and the patient – it may be a compromise at the lowest end of the normal weight range. A weight-gaining diet is also agreed, usually based on eating a set number of calories, starting with around 1500 and increasing gradually to about 3000 a day. Calorie counting is second nature to most anorectic people; it reassures them that they are not being stuffed full indiscriminately and allows them to feel in control of the weight gain. Problems and feelings experienced during meals should be noted in the diaries, for discussion later. Making a big deal of mealtime problems when they happen puts unhelpful pressure on sufferers when they feel most vulnerable.

Refeeding, as doctors call it, is essential to reverse real starvation. It is not always necessary: some sufferers turn up for help before becoming that ill. Refeeding is not always entirely voluntary, either. Severely anorectic patients may have to be fed at first by liquid food through drips into their veins or through nasal tubes leading into their stomachs. Others may have to be watched all the time, during and after meals that may take an hour or more, to make sure that they do not throw away or throw up the food. Serious starvation is a kind of suicide attempt, just as much as taking an overdose: if an anorectic person refuses to go to hospital it may occasionally become necessary for her to be admitted compulsorily, or 'sectioned', under the Mental Health Act (see Chapter 9).

Drugs are used occasionally in treating anorexia nervosa. Antipsychotic drugs like chlorpromazine (Largactil), usually used for illnesses like schizophrenia, stimulate appetite as a side effect. They also treat the transient psychotic symptoms, like delusions and hallucinations, that probably occur in the small percentage of anorectic people who also have borderline personality disorder. Antidepressants can help for sufferers who are also depressed.

Psychological therapy is the other important component of treatment; it includes behaviour therapy, counselling and psychotherapy. Behaviour therapy is used to change patterns of abnormal eating and losing weight. Firstly, behaviour modification programmes that reward acceptable behaviour (see p. 127 for basic principles) are often used during refeeding treatment. The abnormal patterns of behaviour, detailed in patients' eating diaries, are gradually replaced by three meals a day without vomiting, purging, or exercise. Secondly, cognitive behaviour therapy may be used in the longer term to challenge and alter anorectic ways of thinking (for basic principles see pp. 74–5).

Counselling, or at a more intense level, psychotherapy, are aimed at helping sufferers to feel better about themselves. The general themes which tend to underlie anorexia nervosa are explored along with any special reasons why it started, perhaps leaving home. Anorectic patients who still live with their parents often need help with their whole families, in family therapy. For those who have managed to leave home and separate from their parents, one-to-one therapy is probably better.

Parents usually feel particularly vulnerable and guilty when their children develop anorexia nervosa. Although it might have started because of difficulties in family relationships, no one is suggesting that parents should blame themselves. Those parents who want help in coping and do not get enough support from friends and family can talk to their GPs and to the specialists involved. Many parents feel excluded from decisions and plans during their children's treatment. But this exclusion may be for good reasons, because anorexia nervosa often arises from lack of self-control over growing up, low self-esteem, and problems with learning how to live responsibly. The Eating Disorders Association understands parents' experiences and can offer advice and support to them.

Outcome in Anorexia Nervosa

Treatment for anorexia nervosa in a specialized hospital unit takes three months on average. Urgent physical treatment and refeeding usually work. But keeping anorectic people well for the rest of their lives is much harder and much less successful. The American Psychiatric Association produced guidelines in 1993 on treating eating disorders and said that only one-half of sufferers have completely recovered after four years. About a quarter improve but still have anorectic attitudes, and a quarter remain severely underweight with period problems. The last group may still improve over the next few years but recovery after about 10 years is rare. About 3% of anorectics die in the first 10 years of the illness – half of them commit suicide, mostly by taking overdoses.

Jane, who was described earlier, was luckier. After her overdose she spent three months in a special psychiatric unit. It took her several weeks to trust the staff and believe that they would help her gain weight very slowly. Her periods started again, in a haphazard way at first. Eventually she regained her weight and her old personality, and could see that she had got into a bad way. A year after her overdose things became stormy at home again. But this time the rows were because Jane had a boyfriend and wanted to stay out late – a much happier kind of problem that was eventually solved by a much more adult kind of negotiation.

BULIMIA NERVOSA

This is an eating disorder related to anorexia nervosa. The biggest difference between the two conditions (see Box 4) is that people with bulimia nervosa have impulsive binges of massive overeating followed by self-induced vomiting or excessive purging using laxatives.

BOX 4

	Comparison between bulimia nervosa and anorexia nervosa	
	Bulimia	*Anorexia*
Onset	14–40 years	14–25 years
Psychology	Fear of fatness	Fear of normal weight
Weight before	Normal or high	Normal
Weight after	Normal or high	Low
Behaviour	Dieting, bingeing, vomiting, purging	Dieting, vomiting, purging, exercising
Periods	Irregular or normal	Stopped
Fatal	Rarely	In 3 out of 100

Bulimia nervosa tends to affect women from about 16 to 40, and one-quarter of sufferers are married. Although it involves very strange behaviour and can be dangerous sometimes, and although some sufferers have anorexia nervosa too, bulimia nervosa does not usually lead to serious starvation. Weight is often normal.

About 1–2% of young women in Britain have bulimia nervosa. Occasional episodes of binge eating and vomiting seem to be much commoner, particularly in certain groups: among college students up to 15% of women and 5% of men admit to having bulimic symptoms at some time. A study in Switzerland, however, found that only 4% of people in their late twenties who were picked randomly from the general population were binge eaters, two-thirds of them women.[3] One in five of the whole group, however, were worried about their weight and one in ten were on diets even though hardly any of them were actually overweight. Of the dieters, most were women. Of the few overweight people, most were men. Bulimia nervosa among men has been noted by several groups of researchers, in contrast with anorexia nervosa, which affects men extremely rarely.

Symptoms of Bulimia Nervosa

Physical Symptoms

Binge eating is the main physical feature of bulimia nervosa. Typical binges are huge and uncontrolled, often comprising odd things like a whole raw cabbage, a loaf of bread, and an entire packet of cereal, at one sitting. Sufferers have been known to consume as much as 40,000 calories in a day – more than 20 times the normal energy requirement for an average sized woman. Between binges most sufferers diet strictly; some even fast. All the abnormal eating is done in secrecy.

Soon after binge eating, sufferers nearly always make themselves sick, often by poking their fingers down their throats. Many take big doses of laxatives. Not surprisingly, it is bad for the body to vomit so much. The stomach may develop small tears which bleed, and its acid contents may cause burns in the gullet, pits in the teeth, and infection in the salivary glands. The hands of someone with bulimia sometimes show telltale bite marks on the knuckles, made while gagging. Dehydration and mineral imbalances can be dangerous if vomiting persists; loss of potassium can even cause heart attacks.

Bulimia does not interfere with the menstrual cycle unless it is accompanied by anorexia nervosa, when moderate starvation will make periods irregular.

Psychological Problems

People with bulimia are much more like the average dieter than people with anorexia nervosa: not necessarily thin and sometimes a bit overweight. Like most dieters, they want to avoid fatness. In many this amounts to a strong fear of fatness. Most do not, however, have the abnormal perception of body size that occurs in anorexia nervosa.

Some people with bulimia say that a binge can block out unpleasant emotions in the same way that alcohol can. But binge eating makes most sufferers feel bad: intensely guilty, ashamed, and angry with themselves.

In the short term the bad feelings, along with the great

physical discomfort from being so full of food, lead to the desire to vomit. After vomiting sufferers say they feel relieved and often elated. The reasons for this elation are complex, and may be similar to the relief described by people who cut themselves deliberately.

One woman with bulimia described these experiences and feelings graphically in a women's magazine:

> A tight knot of panic adds its painful burden to the pile of half chewed, hastily swallowed food. Beads of perspiration on my brow and my upper lip, as I think of the calories I have stuffed and must now rid myself of. I shove my hand in my mouth and gag, but I have done this so often recently that the natural responses no longer occur. I do not vomit. The food remains, a great mass in my distended belly. My fingernails tear at the back of my throat until it bleeds and my teeth scar the back of my hand, reopening the unhealed blisters from the last binge. I catch sight of my face in the mirror – pale, shining skin, gaping mouth, desperate, bulging eyes pouring useless tears. Saliva runs down my chin and up my arm; still I do not vomit.
>
> I've read about bulimics so practised in their art that they can vomit spontaneously. In my worst moments I envy those women. Finally, it starts to come out, in little heaps, or sometimes in a great gush. Sore on a raw throat, sore on the belly that's been contracting and convulsing. But what a relief to the mind! Relax. It's over. The bloated stomach is empty, the hands shaky and the legs weak, but the conscience is fleetingly free. The regurgitated contents of an entire carrier bag are flushed away now, and no one knows what I have done, because it doesn't show. I'll never let it show.
>
> I've filled the void nicely and I'll deal with my problems – finance, relationships, unfulfilled ambitions – tomorrow. Because I won't binge then. I'll be a different woman in the morning, strong and determined.[4]

Causes of Bulimia Nervosa

Risk Factors
There has not been much research on the underlying causes of bulimia nervosa. In essence, it is an abnormal extension of dieting which may be brought on by certain additional factors (see Box 5). Around four-fifths of sufferers try to lose weight by dieting before their symptoms start.

BOX 5

Probable causes of bulimia nervosa
Risk factors
Dieting
Family stresses
Social pressures
Other mental health problems
personality disorder, depression, alcohol problems
Past sexual abuse
Triggers for bingeing
Acute stress

Most of the factors linked to anorexia nervosa can also cause bulimia nervosa, although whether inheritance plays a role is not known. One of the less common causes of anorexia nervosa, borderline personality disorder, is thought to be a much bigger factor among bulimic sufferers (detailed on pp. 225–27). Depression and alcohol problems frequently coexist with bulimia.

Another factor that researchers keep finding among people with bulimia, and to a lesser extent in anorexia nervosa, is a history of sexual abuse. Up to half of women with eating disorders say they have been subjected to unwanted sexual experiences in the past; most have bulimia.[5] This may not say anything specific about bulimia: about half of all women admitted to psychiatric hospitals say they have been abused.

Precipitating Factors or Triggers
Whatever the underlying causes of bulimia nervosa, many sufferers say that their binges are triggered by unpleasant emotions like depression, anxiety, and frustration. Impulsive binge eating dispels these feelings at first; then vomiting and purging dispel the secondary emotions aroused by bingeing. The pattern than becomes hard to resist – the only way to feel all right is to go through the whole cycle.

Treatment of Bulimia Nervosa, and its Outcome
Serious physical complications of bulimia nervosa like mineral imbalances have to be corrected in hospital. Psychological treatment follows later.

Behaviour therapy is more effective in stopping the symptoms of bulimia nervosa than psychotherapy based solely on talking. Psychotherapy, however, may be needed by those women whose problems are related to sexual abuse in the past.

As in anorexia nervosa, one of the first steps in behaviour therapy is to keep an eating diary. The diary then provides a basis for altering behaviour. Therapies include anxiety management training (to beat the stressful triggers without having to binge and purge), behaviour modification (explaining and aiming at healthy eating patterns), and cognitive therapy (retraining the mind to challenge and dispel bulimic thoughts). All of these behaviour therapies work. Research studies show that 70–80% of sufferers stop bingeing and vomiting during treatment over three to four months. Cognitive therapy is particularly helpful when sufferers are also depressed.

Antidepressant drugs are also used, particularly fluoxetine (Prozac). This is a member of the new antidepressant group called selective serotonin reuptake inhibitors or SSRIs. It works by increasing brain concentrations of the chemical serotonin, which is thought to be important in regulating mood and controlling eating. Antidepressants help in bulimia in the short term but are less effective than behaviour therapy in the long term.

COMPULSIVE EATING

Culture and fashion affect the way we see our own body shapes, and they also affect our images of others. To most of us obesity means an undesirable degree of fatness, associated with poor physical fitness and unattractiveness. Yet until quite recently, dimply curves were the very essence of beauty for women, as portrayed in many classical paintings of nudes.

BOX 6   Obesity can be defined technically in two ways:

- A weight that is more than one-fifth above the normal range (based on the average weight in the whole population) – by this definition one-fifth of British adults are obese.

- A weight that is too great in comparison with height, as shown by a ratio, the body mass index. This is worked out by dividing a person's weight in kilograms by the square of their height in metres. An index of over 25 indicates obesity. This sounds complicated, but it is common sense that the taller someone is, the more he or she can weigh without being too heavy (and fat). About one-third of adults in Britain are obese by this standard.

Doctors use more technical, less pejorative definitions of obesity (see Box 6). They try to encourage their obese patients to lose weight to avoid a range of related physical problems including heart disease, gall stones, diabetes and complications after operations.

There is still have much to learn, however, about the causes of obesity. Everyone knows anecdotes about fat people who hardly eat a thing, and there is evidence that some may have a deficiency or malfunction of a certain kind of fat cells (brown adipose tissue) in their bodies. But most people who are obese overeat.

Research has not found any general psychological cause for obesity. But some obese people seek help because they do not like themselves, do not cope well socially, or do not feel in control. Organizations such as Weightwatchers can make all the difference – dieting alongside others who feel the same way and who suffer the same problems can be a huge incentive to keep trying. It is also important to exercise regularly.

Some people feel addicted to food. They get stuck in a cycle of dieting alternating with binge eating. In many ways this is bulimia nervosa without the weight-reducing strategies of vomiting and purging. Susie Orbach, a feminist American psychotherapist who now works in London and specializes in helping women with eating disorders, describes a syndrome of compulsive and uncontrolled eating. The features of compulsive eating are summarized in Box 7.

BOX 7

> **Symptoms of compulsive eating**
> - Eating when not physically hungry
> - Feeling out of control around food; dieting or bingeing
> - Often thinking and worrying about food
> - Scouring the latest diet for vital information
> - Feeling awful about yourself as someone who is out of control
> - Feeling awful about your body

Causes of Compulsive Eating
The main cause seems to be preoccupation with body shape, which affects women much more than men because of their

roles in today's Western societies. Susie Orbach says women 'must both blend in and stand out'.

But not all women who worry about body shape are obese. Personal psychological factors are important too. According to Susie Orbach these include underlying and long-term fears of having to compete with other women, which become irrelevant when you're very fat, and much more immediate feelings of anxiety and anger that can be quelled by overeating. In her book *Fat is a Feminist Issue*[6] she explains these and related psychological causes of compulsive eating. She also describes how sufferers can overcome their problems and lose weight without even dieting by getting together in self-help groups (see below).

Treatment of Compulsive Eating
Compulsive eaters who want to break the habit and lose weight effectively can help themselves by keeping eating diaries (see Box 8 for an example).

BOX 8

Time	Food eaten	What I was doing	Feelings before . . .	after
8 a.m.	Coffee only	Getting dressed	Hungry	Pleased
10 a.m.	Coffee and two chocolate bars	Audio typing	Hungry	Fed up
11 a.m.	Crisps	Audio typing	Bored	Fed up
12 noon	Apple	Lunch in canteen	Not hungry	Pleased

Then they can see where they might be going wrong. They should keep the diary, recording honestly what they do, for a couple of weeks before trying to change the pattern of eating. It will probably change before that, but sufferers should not try too hard in this testing period. Once they are quite sure of the pattern they can alter it by using calorie charts to plan weight-reducing meals and by avoiding the triggers that make them overeat. Weightwatchers and other dieting groups offer similar advice and do much to boost confidence and resolve. The Eating Disorders Association, whose address is given in Appendix 2, also offers advice and support.

GPs can help by explaining the problem and the essentials of a healthy diet, setting targets for weight loss, and generally making obese patients feel they have someone else to answer to. They can also make referrals for more specialized help including specialized nutritional advice, cognitive behaviour therapy, and psychotherapy if necessary. Susie Orbach's unit, the Women's Therapy Centre in London, offers private psychotherapy. Its address is given in Appendix 2. People who want to try her therapy for themselves can set up self-help groups based on the detailed advice in *Fat is a Feminist Issue*. The groups work on mutual support, honest talk about eating and being fat, keeping eating diaries, confronting the compulsive eating, and learning how to cope without a psychologically protective layer of fat.

Physical treatments can help obesity but have very little, if any, effect on compulsive eating. Very low calorie diets and slimming pills like fenfluramine do cause weight loss, but they tend to make people lose a lot of fluid which will return during normal eating and do not permanently break the cycle of abnormal eating. They cannot, therefore, guarantee long-term success. For people with extreme obesity who are at great risk of physical complications, for instance, very high blood pressure, drastic measures can be life-saving. These include wiring the jaws together for some weeks or months so that only liquid foods can be taken and stomach surgery to reduce absorption of food. But without additional psychological treatment these measures can be very distressing; a real last resort.

Lifelong Troubles

> There are times when I look over the various parts of my character with perplexity. I recognize that I am made up of several persons and that the person that at the moment has the upper hand will inevitably give place to another. But which is the real one? All of them or none of them?
>
> From *A Writer's Notebook* by W. Somerset Maugham

Personality is one of those words that we all use but find hard to define. It means more or less the same as character. It includes all the features that differentiate each of us as individuals: our traits, habits, attitudes and experiences. Personality can be used to sum up a person's most specific and striking characteristics: 'What's he like?' 'Well, he's got a generous personality.' Or it can be used very generally; someone with 'a lot of personality' is probably sociable and likeable.

Psychologists and psychiatrists trying to define personality usually come up with long-winded explanations like this:

> Personality means the characteristic patterns of behaviour and thought that determine a person's response and adjustment to the world. The concept encompasses temperament (in turn defined as a style of behaviour which includes activity level, emotional reactivity, sociability, impulsivity, aggressivity, and inhibition) as well as intellect, motivation, attitudes, beliefs, and moral values. Characteristic ways of behaving and thinking are called traits and when several traits

commonly occur together they are said to constitute personality types.

With such a huge and imprecise definition it is no wonder that Professor Carl Sandstrom, a child psychologist from Sweden, called the concept of personality scientifically unwieldy and 'one of the most presumptuous terms in modern psychology'.

None the less, psychologists and doctors find personality a useful concept. It can predispose to illness: for instance people whose personalities make them lifetime worriers tend to develop anxiety states under relatively low degrees of stress. It affects the response to illness and some people seem to cope with illness much more easily than others. Personality may even be mistaken for illness: eccentric people are often thought, wrongly, to be mentally ill.

Personality has a powerful influence right through life. One consultant in old-age psychiatry in London always reminds her staff not to assume that elderly patients' difficult behaviour is necessarily down to illness: it may just be plain awkwardness. Forgetting that old people have personalities is a common mistake, and one that can be quite patronizing.

It is easy to forget that personality is important right at the start of life, too. Newborn babies may look alike, but they vary a lot in things like level of activity, attention span, adaptability to changes in the environment and general mood. And many of these early features persist, becoming part of the adult personality. There is a two-way relationship between these inborn characteristics and life's experiences: if you behave in a certain way, you will be treated by others in a certain way. This kind of reinforcement and moulding of personality traits continues through life. For example, an outgoing person will, quite literally, go out more than a shy person and thereby become even more sociable.

This combination of nature and nurture, however, does not always work well. Some people develop personalities that are troublesome to themselves, or others, or both. They may be odd, or unlikeable, or badly behaved. If personality causes big and long-lasting trouble, enough to come to the attention of a doctor, it may attract the psychiatric label of personality disorder.

PERSONALITY DISORDERS

Psychiatrists use the term personality disorders to describe persistently odd or antisocial behaviour problems that do not quite amount to recognizable mental illness. The term is almost exclusively used by psychiatrists. Behaving strangely enough to attract psychiatric attention is almost essential to the diagnosis. This kind of behaviour includes repeated self-harm without being depressed and violence to others without being sorry or insane. Of course, many people who might be called personality disordered if referred to psychiatrists end up in the criminal justice system – often in prison.

When non-psychiatrists (mainly other doctors and health professionals, the police and courts, and the affected people's relatives) are faced with behaviour like repeated overdosing they often think, quite reasonably, that the behaviour must be caused by mental illness. But mental illness tends to have definite symptoms that differ pretty clearly from the experiences and feelings that sufferers have when well. If a person who previously seemed completely normal (whatever that means) suddenly begins to behave abnormally he or she may be ill. If, however, the person's behaviour has always been abnormal and has simply worsened then the problem may lie in the personality.

Personality disorders do not have clear-cut symptoms. They are thought to be an intrinsic part of the personality, making people who have them more or less permanently different from the rest of society. Personality disorder, therefore, is a social definition.

The international classification of diseases that is used by doctors in Britain calls personality disorders 'basic faults in personal functioning that give rise to ingrained and maladaptive behaviour, attitudes, and emotional responses which cause suffering to the self or others and are associated with social impairment'. Other, shorter psychiatric definitions include 'persistent, pervasive abnormalities in social relationships and social functioning generally' and 'abnormal personalities who suffer through their abnormalities and through whose abnormalities society suffers'.

In a detailed critique of the concept of personality disorder three psychiatrists have pointed out what a judgmental diagnosis it is:

> . . . personality disorder must always be judged by its effects on others, be they friends, relations or others in close contact with the patient, or society as a whole. Society thereby imposes its own yardstick on the definition of personality disorder . . . Using [the] definition literally, Heinrich Himmler and Hermann Goering had normal personalities between 1933 and 1943, and Andre Sakharov and Nelson Mandela are personality disordered, since they have caused suffering to themselves and others through trying to reform the widest manifestation of society, the state.[1]

Two other psychiatrists have suggested that personality disorder is a pejorative label that allows psychiatrists to reject difficult patients.[2] The article's authors asked about one in eight of all British qualified psychiatrists to read a description of a patient and explain (by completing a detailed questionnaire) how they would diagnose and treat him. The basic history described a young man with financial problems who complained of depression and suicidal feelings. He had taken an overdose of tablets two years earlier and had been seen by a psychiatrist who diagnosed a personality disorder. Recently, the man had been taking sleeping pills for insomnia and he now seemed reluctant to give them up, according to his GP. Some of the psychiatrists in the survey were asked to comment on this history, others were sent versions that differed slightly. In one version the patient was a woman, in another the patient's occupation (a solicitor) was mentioned, in another no previous diagnosis was given, and in the last the previous diagnosis was depression. The first version prompted the least sympathetic responses. This seemed to confirm the authors' theory that a previous diagnosis of personality disorder encourages psychiatrists to make negative value judgements about patients and take them less seriously.

But Tyrer and colleagues point out in their article that personality disorder is a useful diagnosis. It is common (being applicable to up to 13% of the general population and as much as 70% of the prison population), deeply disturbing, and a big part of psychiatric practice. Personality disorders are said to affect at least half of all people who take non-fatal overdoses and harm themselves in other non-lethal ways like wrist cutting (see Chapter 9 for more detail on self-harm).

The reason psychiatrists might want to avoid such patients, however, is that personality disorders are very difficult and sometimes impossible to treat. And the people who have them can be, by definition, absolutely infuriating. They reject help and sympathy and do not seem to want to help themselves. Yet saying that someone has a personality disorder, not a mental illness, implies that he or she bears some responsibility for the odd or antisocial behaviour. Carol's story is fairly typical:

Carol would be ready for discharge from hospital in a few days. Her broken ankle and arm were doing well, and her liver was functioning properly again. The nurses on the ward could not understand why the psychiatrists had refused to transfer Carol to their unit – this poor girl must need something more than an outpatient appointment, surely? After all, she must have meant to kill herself; nobody who wants to survive takes an overdose and jumps out of a window. And she had tried to kill herself before, apparently.

Carol certainly did not enjoy life. In the past 10 years she had taken 16 overdoses; several of them while in a psychiatric hospital. She had twice broken a leg, once by running out in front of a car and once by jumping in front of a slow-moving train.

Carol was 32. She lived with her elderly parents, who

devoted their lives to worrying about her but got nowhere with her. She barely spoke to them or her married sister and she had no friends. Her last job, as a shelf filler in a supermarket, had been more than two years ago. Yet she had been bright at school and had been expected to go on to college.

Psychiatrists had tried everything to help Carol and had failed miserably. The first of her many admissions to psychiatric hospital was at 17 after she took an overdose of aspirin tablets. Then, as now, it was hard to understand what Carol was feeling. She rarely talked to other patients or to staff, and answered most questions about herself with a vague 'I don't know', or a bland 'I'm fine'. She said that her relationship with her parents was fine, too. She seemed sulky and bored, and chose to spend much of the day on her bed, apparently asleep. She did not seem particularly sad, hopeless, or distressed, although she was often irritable. On several occasions Carol screamed at some of the older patients, particularly one elderly woman whom she assaulted twice by kicking and punching her.

Carol's behaviour, her apparent indifference to life, and her lack of clear symptoms perplexed and worried her psychiatrist. So he kept Carol in hospital for nearly a year and tried her unsuccessfully on numerous treatments – psychotherapy, tranquillizers (to which she later became addicted), antidepressants, lithium, depot injections, and even ECT (electroconvulsive therapy). Carol was not kept in hospital against her will: she didn't seem to care where she lived.

During a later admission Carol was referred to the hospital's group psychotherapy unit – a special facility called a therapeutic community. The psychiatric team and the psychotherapist who had tried individual therapy with Carol hoped that group therapy might help her relate to others and, perhaps, to explore her feelings about herself and her family. But it wasn't a success. Carol was unable or unwilling to look at her problems:

she said that was fine and that everyone else had problems that made the world a hostile place. For two months Carol arrived late at group therapy sessions, walked out of them early, and frequently shouted at other members of the community for boring her. Eventually, they voted her out because she showed no desire to change and was too disruptive.

During the first couple of admissions to hospital Carol was diagnosed as having an unusual form of depression. Despite the lack of definite depressive symptoms, her clear distaste for life made the diagnosis seem reasonable. And there must have been something wrong, for her to behave like that. But her intent to kill herself was never convincing. She always took a sub-lethal dose of pills (and on one occasion, weed killer) and immediately told someone what she had done. Over the years her problems were so persistent, so unresponsive to treatment and, apparently, so intrinsic to her life that the diagnosis changed to one of personality disorder. There seemed to be little that anyone could do except wait for Carol to kill herself one day.

Over the years British and European psychiatrists have come up with several subtypes of personality disorder. These include terms like obsessional, paranoid, explosive, and hysterical – all self-explanatory names. American psychiatrists use a simpler classification with just three broad headings: eccentric (odd and withdrawn), dramatic (antisocial and attention seeking), and fearful (unable to cope well with life). Most British psychiatrists have stopped using the full range of separate labels, however, and just use the general term. Only one subtype is used now: borderline personality disorder (which is more or less the same thing as the legal term psychopathic disorder – see Chapter 9). It was first used in the US, as an example of the dramatic kind of personality disorder.

Borderline Personality Disorder or Psychopathic Disorder

People with borderline personality disorder are thought to suffer very transient but considerably disturbing symptoms of mental illness. The symptoms may last only a day – long enough to prompt an often dramatic and violent reaction – but not long enough to amount to full-blown illness. Hence the term borderline: sufferers hover on the edge of illness and occasionally slip into it. Having these symptoms on top of an abnormal personality seems to make people with this disorder particularly difficult to deal with, often because they are threatening and violent. Alan's story illustrates this:

> The magistrate wasn't sure what to make of Alan. Clearly, he was dangerous and should be locked up. Only 28, he had been in prison four times already and it seemed to have little effect on him. Most of his previous convictions were for violence, including attacks on his widowed mother, whom he had terrorized for many years. This time, the magistrate decided to remand Alan in prison for psychiatric assessment before passing sentence.
>
> Alan was not overtly mentally ill. His offence was, sadly, common enough: he had assaulted an old woman. But he hadn't had any obvious motive. Although he had broken into the woman's home, Alan had made no attempt to take anything. Instead he had beaten her badly in her bed. She was deaf and had not heard Alan entering the house while she slept.
>
> Alan showed no remorse when he was interviewed by the psychiatrist. He said that he had attacked the woman because he had seen her many times in the local shops and had been annoyed by her loud voice (she did not wear a hearing aid and tended to shout). He was easily annoyed, he said.
>
> The psychiatrist later told the court that Alan was a tense, immature person who reacted to stress with outbursts of paranoia and aggression and showed a complete disregard for other people's feelings. His para-

noia was always directed against women. He firmly believed that they all found him repulsive and threatening and he hated them vehemently for it. Some of them, like the woman he attacked, really had it in for him and tried to provoke him, he said. Alan freely admitted to the psychiatrist that he would probably attack women again in future.

The psychiatrist explained that, although Alan was not mentally ill, he had a persistent problem in his attitude to women. When this was exaggerated by a stressful incident – even something as minor as irritation at a loud voice – Alan became briefly deluded and paranoid. This might be alleviated or, at least, prevented from worsening, in hospital. The psychiatrist said Alan had borderline personality disorder. He recommended that Alan should be admitted compulsorily to a secure (i.e. locked and guarded) psychiatric unit under the Mental Health Act.

Mainstream psychiatry did not recognize until the 1980s that personality disorders could include transient but powerful symptoms, like Alan's paranoia. Before borderline personality disorder was coined, British psychiatrists used the term psychopathic personality to explain the behaviour of non-juvenile delinquents who were severely and persistently antisocial but were not simply mad or bad. People with this problem were called psychopaths. This is much narrower than the non-medical definition of psychopath, which tends to be used for anyone who is mentally ill and overtly disturbed – perhaps because it gets confused with the term psychotic. Another non-medical word, criminality, is probably much closer to the idea of psychopathic or borderline personality disorder.

Although psychiatry has sharpened up its terminology as it has discovered more about the experiences of such people, the legal system has not. The law which authorizes compulsory assessment and treatment of certain mentally ill people, the Mental Health Act 1983 (England and Wales), still uses the term psychopathic disorder (see Chapter 9). The Act calls it 'a persistent disorder or disability of mind (whether or not including significant impairment of intelligence) which results in abnormally aggressive or seriously irresponsible conduct on the part of the person concerned'. This may seem much like the everyday psychiatric definition, but the law adds a further dimension – treatability. For a compulsory treatment order to be made on the grounds of psychopathic disorder, there must be evidence that treatment is 'likely to alleviate or prevent a deterioration of the condition'. Whether or not psychopathic disorder (or borderline personality disorder) and the other personality disorders are treatable is discussed later (see p. 231).

Causes of Personality Disorders

Nobody knows for sure what makes some people odd or antisocial. There is no single causative factor but there is some evidence that inheritance, changes in the brain, upbringing, and social conditioning all play a part (see Box 1).

BOX 1	**Possible causes of personality disorder**
	• Inheritance
	• Changes in the brain
	• Upbringing and childhood problems
	• Social conditioning

Inheritance
There has not been much genetic research on personality disorder, but there has been plenty on criminality, mostly in twins.[3] This persistent tendency to commit crimes has been found to occur twice as often in both twins of a pair when they are identical than when they are non-identical. It is reasonable to assume that both halves of twin pairs will get similar upbringings, whether or not they are genetically identical. Therefore, when some attribute occurs more

commonly in identical twins it is probably produced by their genes rather than by something in their shared home environment.

Criminality is much commoner in men than women. This is probably because women's other personality features and roles in society give them more control over themselves than the same factors do in men. In other words, women have a higher threshold than men for committing crimes and those women who do become persistent criminals probably have very strong genetic tendencies to criminality. Studies of criminal female twins bear out this theory.

Another theory is that criminality is inherited mainly on the male sex chromosome (the Y chromosome) and is, therefore, very common among men with a rare abnormality that gives them two Y chromosomes instead of one (the so-called XYY men). This theory arose from the observation that an unusually high proportion of male inmates in a hospital for mentally ill offenders had XYY chromosomes. But further work has shown that this abnormality tends to make men big and tall with below average IQs, factors that can make them seem (when arrested) particularly threatening and in need of treatment in a secure hospital. Men with XYY in the general population are not unusually criminal, and the Y chromosome may not be the culprit.

The genetics of criminality probably explain something of how borderline or psychopathic personality disorder is inherited. And studies on criminality are backed up by the few on personality disorders. For example, research on people with psychopathic disorder who were adopted in infancy shows that their biological or natural relatives are much more likely to have the same disorder than are their adoptive relatives.

Changes in the Brain

Electroencephalograms (EEG brainwave tests) done in the 1950s and 60s on people with antisocial and aggressive behaviour found that about two-thirds had abnormal brainwaves. The brainwave patterns suggested that the brains had not fully matured during growing up. In theory, genetic abnormalities could slow down brain development in people who grow up with borderline personality disorders. This has not, however, been confirmed.

Upbringing and Childhood Behavioural Problems

In the 1940s it was thought that children who were separated from their mothers, perhaps by death or by going into children's homes, were particularly likely to become aggressive and criminal in adolescence and adulthood. This has not been borne out by more recent research. But it is true, perhaps unsurprisingly, that children with seriously antisocial behaviour are more likely than others to be antisocial adults.

In the 1970s Professor Michael Rutter, a child psychiatrist, studied more than 2000 schoolchildren in the Isle of Wight as 10-year-olds and again at 14. He and his team found that only a fifth had persistent psychological problems at 14 and that fewer than one-twelfth had definite psychiatric disorders. Thus, most of the teenagers studied were not significantly disturbed. Most of those who were had behavioural problems called conduct disorders.

Conduct disorder is the term used by child psychiatrists to describe persistently antisocial behaviour (such as truancy, stealing, or aggression) that is more than simple naughtiness or disobedience. The term is only applied when psychiatric problems such as anxiety and depression, which can disrupt behaviour, have been ruled out. It may seem unnecessary to provide a psychiatric label for children's antisocial behaviour. After all, it often seems an understandable reaction to an unhappy life: conduct disorders occur most commonly among boys from families with many social and domestic problems. But psychiatrists may be asked to assess such children, and the use of a label makes their task easier. Other doctors such as GPs will understand the shorthand term, and parents may feel that a label is easier to come to terms with than a diagnosis of: 'Well, there's something wrong which will probably persist, but it isn't actually an illness and there isn't really a specific treatment.'

Another more familiar label is juvenile delinquency. Technically, this term is used only by lawyers, not psychiatrists, and is applied to children and teenagers with repeated and serious criminal convictions. Nearly all teenage boys admit to law-breaking when asked directly, and this is an old problem that goes back even to Shakespeare's time:

> I would there were no age between sixteen and three-and-twenty, or that youth would sleep out the rest; for there is nothing in the between but getting wenches with child, wronging the ancientry, stealing, fighting.
> From *The Winter's Tale* by William Shakespeare

Most teenagers, however, commit trivial offences and only a tenth are convicted more than once. Most are not delinquents. Most teenagers grow out of rebelliousness, disobedience, and minor offending as they learn to assert their independence and authority in more constructive ways. But some of those who have behaved badly enough to attract labels of conduct disorder and delinquency will keep them into adulthood.

Social Conditioning
Whatever the underlying causes of antisocial behaviour, it is likely to persist and become ingrained if it is reinforced through life. Part of this reinforcement may come from the family. Perhaps other members of the family behave badly too, setting poor examples. And perhaps some parents are less interested in or successful at laying down family rules than others. Finally, antisocial behaviour may be reinforced because it has certain advantages – it draws attention and it can mask emotional problems that are too hard to deal with directly.

These social theories may all ring true. But they have not been extensively researched yet. For a review of these and other theories of causation for personality disorders see the *Oxford Textbook of Psychiatry*.[4]

Treatment for Personality Disorders

Are personality disorders treatable? By definition, the answer should be 'no'. Personality disorders are diagnosed by excluding recognizable and mostly treatable psychiatric illnesses.

None the less, many people diagnosed as having personality disorders benefit from psychotherapy, as long as they are prepared to work on the idea that their problems come from within.

Because problems with social relations are common in these disorders treatment in a group can be more effective than one-to-one psychotherapy. Therapeutic communities may be particularly helpful. They are places where patients meet together daily and may live together, if the community is in a residential unit or hospital. The structure of the group is democratic, as far as possible. Staff do not wear uniforms and are called by their first names. Patients are encouraged to express themselves freely but must accept that others can confront them with the effects of their words and actions. They must also accept certain communal responsibilities, including decision-making on issues like the admission and discharge of fellow members. For many people who have problems relating to others, this kind of community provides the first chance to really see how they appear to others. This may be a painful experience but may also allow group members to learn that, as well as weaknesses, they have unrecognized strengths that can be built on.

There has been very little research on the outcome of psychological treatment for personality disorders. Studies of former members of therapeutic communities suggest that up to two-thirds improve after one or two years. Whatever the facts, psychotherapy is much less likely to work if the affected person cannot accept the idea of having a troublesome personality and blames circumstances, bad luck, or other people for the problem.

Two other approaches have been tried with variable success. Behaviour therapy that rewards acceptable behaviour and discourages antisocial and undesirable behaviour is sometimes useful. For example, someone admitted to hospital after repeated self-harm would agree on and sign a contract with the ward staff, promising not to harm themselves again while in hospital. Rewards for sticking to the contract might include treats like access to a pool table. But this kind of behaviour modification is often considered unethical.

Lastly, most psychiatric drugs have been tried in treating personality disorders. No clear advantages have emerged from research on this. And anyway, response to something like an antidepressant tends to imply that the diagnosis of personality disorder was wrong and that the person had an unusual kind of depression all along. This is when the concept of personality disorder as a real diagnosis looks most shaky.

Treatment for Borderline or Psychopathic Personality Disorder

The law assumes that psychopathic disorder can respond to treatment, because it includes treatability in the criteria for applying the Mental Health Act to people with the problem. Is this just wishful thinking? The answer still isn't clear. There is a tendency for psychiatric diagnoses to be revised once treatment has succeeded or failed. Thus, if Alan (who was described earlier on pp. 225–6) learned to respect and like women through psychotherapy and no longer expressed or showed violence, he would probably be rediagnosed. As with all personality disorders, lack of response to treatment in borderline or psychopathic disorder is usually part of the original diagnostic process.

Drug treatment, mostly with antipsychotic and antidepressant drugs, may help some people with borderline personality disorders. The most promising results come from trials of antipsychotic drugs like chlorpromazine, given in low doses to treat brief psychotic episodes. Lithium, anti-epilepsy drugs, and electroconvulsive therapy (ECT) have also been tried with variable success. There are no clear answers yet. Many more studies will have to be done.

Other Problems Related to Personality Disorders

Two conditions with dramatic features are thought to be related to personality disorders: Munchausen's syndrome and multiple personality disorder.

Munchausen's Syndrome

This problem is named after Baron von Munchausen, a fictitious character who made up very tall stories. People with Munchausen's syndrome fake illness, presumably to get attention. Typically, they tour the country being admitted to a series of hospitals under different false names. They usually simulate illness with great knowledge and skill, choosing specific symptoms that need urgent admission and intervention, often surgery. As soon as the absence of genuine physical illness is realized – and that can take several days if the patient is sufficiently clued up about the assumed symptoms – the patient walks out.

Though psychiatrists are frequently called in such cases, the patients rarely wait to see them, and when they do the diagnosis is usually a personality disorder. Some people with the syndrome fake psychiatric illness and make up long, sad histories of being orphaned or raped. Short-term attention is the only apparent motive. Offers of counselling, housing, and social support are usually rejected. There has been very little research on this syndrome, not least because the people with it do not stay put long enough to be studied.

One rare variant is Munchausen's syndrome by proxy, in which a parent or other carer fakes signs of illness in a child. The motive, theoretically, is to gain indirect attention and sympathy for the parent or carer. One published case report described a child who was thought to have kidney disease until the blood in its urine was tested and found to be the mother's: she had been adding it to the samples. Munchausen's syndrome by proxy gained notoriety in 1993 when Beverley Allitt, a children's nurse who murdered several children in her care, was said to suffer from it.

Multiple Personality Syndrome
This is a very rare but well-publicized problem in which the sufferer seems to have a least two separate personalities, each with a different name and different way of thinking, speaking and behaving. Careful study of sufferers suggests that they make up their second (or multiple) personalities to get attention, although this may not be entirely deliberate and conscious.[5] The cause is thought to be extreme distress over a long period: some researchers have found that as many as 90% of sufferers have been sexually abused in the past. Psychotherapy is the recommended treatment, although some psychiatrists believe that the phenomenon is largely a creation of inexpert psychotherapy.

8 SUICIDE

Ending the Heart-Ache

> To be, or not to be – that is the question;
> Whether 'tis nobler in the mind to suffer
> The slings and arrows of outrageous fortune,
> Or to take arms against a sea of troubles,
> And by opposing end them? To die, to sleep –
> No more; and by a sleep to say we end
> The heart-ache and the thousand natural shocks
> That flesh is heir to. 'Tis a consummation
> Devoutly to be wish'd.
> From *Hamlet* (III, i, 56) by William Shakespeare

Hamlet was not sure which was the nobler response to his troubles; to put up with them or to escape them by suicide. Most societies have no doubt which is nobler and have social, moral and religious objections to suicide. Some even outlaw it.

To individuals the issue may be less clear. There can be few experiences more powerful and frightening than feeling suicidal, yet death can bring relief from unbearable suffering. And for the families and friends left behind, society's apparently clear position on suicide offers little support. Nobody wants to talk about it: the subject is taboo.

Suicide is an uncommon way to die in Britain, accounting for less than one in a hundred of all deaths. Of the 2500 patients on a typical GP's list, one, on average, will die by suicide every three years. But since 1960 apparent attempts at suicide have become all too common. They now account for about 100,000 admissions to Britain's general hospitals each year – a tenth of all acute medical (as opposed to surgical) admissions. Among women admitted to medical wards self-poisoning, usually with a drugs overdose, is the prime emergency. Among men it is second only to heart disease. Staff working in hospital casualty departments typically see two or three survivors of self-poisoning or other deliberate self-harm each day. Among the many emergencies due to problems like heart attacks, strokes and diabetes these patients may seem an unnecessary and unwelcome addition to the workload.

Research shows that fewer than one-sixth of people who harm themselves non-fatally have mental illnesses. And two-thirds admit that they did not intend to kill themselves. Because of this their behaviour is often called parasuicide or deliberate self-harm rather than attempted suicide.

Although most people who harm themselves in this way are not ill they do usually need some kind of help, both physical and psychological. They and their relatives may be extremely distressed after the event. They may need professional help to understand what led up to it. And, more importantly, up to one-third may harm themselves again unless the cause is removed. People who harm themselves are 100 times more likely than the rest of the population to kill themselves in the next year.

About half of the people who actually kill themselves have not tried to do so before and, in many ways, 'successful suicides' tend to differ from 'unsuccessful attempters'.

Causes of Suicide

For those left behind, the family and friends, suicide usually feels an intensely personal act. But suicide does not seem to be caused by internal conflict alone. Annual statistics suggest that certain social and environmental factors affect the number, timing and manner of suicides and dictate to some extent who performs them. The main social and personal factors that probably explain suicide are summarized in Box 1 and described below. These are, however, just guides to what happens because the statistics may be inaccurate. Some suicides do not make it into the statistical reports because they are never proven and are misrecorded as accidental or 'open' verdicts.

BOX 1   **Suicide and Psychiatric Disorder**

Retrospective studies of people who kill themselves show that 90% had a psychiatric problem of some kind:

- 50% were depressed
- 25% had alcohol or drug problems
- 5% had schizophrenia
- The remaining 10% had stress-related problems such as anxiety and panic disorder or had personality disorders – probably undiagnosed, and therefore difficult to confirm retrospectively

---

Social and Environmental Causes

TIME OF YEAR

Overall suicide rates fluctuate from decade to decade, and also show seasonal variations. For unknown reasons suicide occurs most frequently in late spring – in April, May and June in the Northern hemisphere and October, November and December in the South.

This may have something to do with an illness called seasonal affective disorder, in which bouts of depression occur in winter (see p. 69). Even people who do not have the full version of this disorder may feel particularly gloomy in winter, too gloomy and flat to consider anything as angry and forceful as suicide. Suicide may happen more in the spring because depressive feelings are still present but sufferers start to feel stimulated and active.

MALE UNEMPLOYMENT

Men are more likely to commit suicide than women. Over the past 20 years in Britain the suicide rate for women has fallen while that for men has risen, particularly in the highlands of Scotland. During the two world wars relatively few men killed themselves (perhaps because so many were killed by war) but between the wars, in the 1930's economic depression when many men were unemployed, the rate shot up.

Mass unemployment may explain why the suicide rate among young men (aged 15–24) in Britain has risen by 75% since 1982 and is now second only to accidents as this age group's commonest cause of death. The rate is particularly high where mass unemployment has persisted and has affected two or even three generations. In these areas society is very different from that in more prosperous places: unemployment creates an atmosphere of hopelessness and pointlessness which probably makes young men who are already vulnerable more likely to feel suicidal. This echoes the theories of Emile Durkheim, a French social philosopher at the turn of the century, who said that all suicide was an expression of the disintegration of society. Similar patterns have occurred in other European countries that have also suffered high unemployment over the past two decades.[1]

ACCESS TO METHODS OF SUICIDE

The ways in which people kill themselves vary from country to country, mainly because the availability of lethal weapons and substances varies. For example, it is no surprise that suicide using a firearm is much commoner in the United States than in Britain.

Methods of suicide also vary within countries over time. In Britain from the early 1920s most houses were supplied with coal gas, which contained highly poisonous carbon monoxide. Its toxicity was well known and, until the changeover to harmless North Sea gas in the 1960s, gassing was twice as common as any other method of suicide. Poisoning using prescribed drugs then took over (initially barbiturates, then benzodiazepine tranquillizers and antidepressants).

Since the 1970s, when safer psychiatric drugs were developed, deaths by poisoning have tailed off again. But overdoses still cause two-thirds of suicides among women. Violent suicide by hanging and drowning is increasing now, particularly among young men. And asphyxiation by car exhaust fumes is now the cause of death in a third of all suicides among men. This will probably start to decline again soon, however, because the amount of carbon monoxide permitted in exhaust emissions from new cars is now tightly controlled.

Personal Causes of Suicide
These social and environmental factors seem to affect overall rates of suicide quite powerfully. But they are huge generalizations, and they do not say much about why people decide to kill themselves.

The most likely Briton to commit suicide is a divorced man, over 40, who lives alone. Chronic stresses such as unhappy retirement or unemployment will increase his risk and so will illness, particularly mental illness. More than 90% of suicides are thought to have suffered from some kind of mental disorder (see Box 2), mostly depression and problems with alcohol and drugs.

BOX 2

Probable causes of suicide

Social and environmental factors
● Time of year
● Male unemployment
● Access to methods of suicide

Personal factors
● Mental disorders
● Long-term stresses
● Brain chemistry (serotonin deficiency)

The remaining 10% may have made considered and rational decisions to die because they had long-term stresses and problems that were insurmountable – progressive physical disease, financial ruin, or failed relationships. Sigmund Freud said that people like these succumbed to a natural death instinct, but later theorists have not agreed with him. More probably, many of them simply overdid parasuicide.

Peter's story illustrates a common path to suicide:

Peter knew that he had hit rock bottom when he phoned the Samaritans. The woman at the other end of the phone hadn't said much, but she had listened to him for 40 minutes. It had taken him almost that long to say how he felt.

Nine months earlier Peter had been made redundant from his job as an architect. He was not the only one to go. The recession had hit the building industry very hard and the knock-on effect to his own profession was quick. But he felt that he had fared particularly badly after applying unsuccessfully for 15 jobs, some of which would have meant demotion.

On the face of it, things might have been worse. Peter's finances were adequate because he had investments, his wife's income from her full-time job as a nurse, and no mortgage (he had paid off the small remainder with his redundancy settlement). He need not have been idle; for years he had wanted time to finish a book that he was writing on the history of art.

But Peter felt useless, hopeless and literally redundant. He couldn't bear the fact that his wife, Jean, had gone back to full-time work after 20 years, even though she seemed to relish it. He felt he had failed his son of 14, who he had had to take out of boarding school and send to the local comprehensive. And, because he hadn't told his elderly mother that he was out of work, Peter hated himself for lying.

For several weeks Peter had felt increasingly depressed. He felt that he was slipping into a deep, dark hole. His guilt and self-blame about redundancy were compounded by a new problem: drinking too much. He had always appreciated good whisky, but was now drinking half a bottle a day and finding it hard to do without. It was affecting his appetite, his sleep, and his concentration. But he couldn't stop. Being drunk at least allowed him to drift away from his unbearable life for a while. Peter had not discussed any of this with Jean, although she noticed that he looked tired and that he was barely eating. She had tried, unsuccessfully, to help him to talk. Jean knew nothing about the alcohol. Peter hid it from her and ate strong mints to disguise the smell of it on his breath before her return from work each day.

Peter wasn't very good at talking, particularly about himself. But, one morning after Jean had left for work, he felt he would burst if he didn't tell someone what was happening to him. He phoned the Samaritans. At least it spared him the shame of talking to someone who knew him. He talked for a long time, and although he couldn't really make himself clear, he felt some relief. But the relief didn't last.

A week later Jean returned from work and heard the car engine running in the locked garage. Peter had sealed the door and window with tape, run a hose into his car from the exhaust pipe, and asphyxiated himself. At the inquest the coroner recorded a verdict of death by suicide. The local paper avoided the word, but reported how Peter died and said that there were no suspicious circumstances.

Most research on the causes of suicide has focused on patterns of behaviour and has come up with stories like Peter's. Recently, however, researchers have looked at what actually brings on suicidal behaviour: what happens in the brain. Understanding the process might lead to a treatment; an anti-suicide pill, perhaps.

Scientists think that a brain chemical called serotonin or

5HT usually suppresses parts of the brain that would, if unchecked, cause impulsive and violent behaviour. If serotonin levels fall, such behaviour is more likely to happen. Low concentrations of serotonin have been found in the brains of people who died by violent suicide and around the spinal cords of people who have committed impulsive murders. This theory is backed up by unrelated research on whether anti-cholesterol drugs reduce deaths from heart disease: the drugs do reduce heart attacks but they actually seem to increase deaths from suicide, accidents and violence.[2] The probable explanation for this is that cholesterol and serotonin have closely related functions in the brain; when cholesterol concentration falls, so does serotonin concentration.

Preventing Suicide

Suicide can be prevented. But prevention is not easy, and it involves many different approaches. In 1992 the British Government made suicide reduction a major target in its strategy to improve everyone's health. Its plan, called the Health of the Nation, named five key areas in which the NHS's efforts to prevent disease would be increased. The five were coronary heart disease and strokes, cancers, mental illness, accidents, and problems related to sexual health including AIDS.

Within each key area the government set specific targets to improve the nation's health. Two of the three targets for improving mental health were about suicide prevention (see Box 3).

BOX 3	**Government targets for improving the nation's mental health by the year 2000**
	• To improve significantly the health and social functioning of mentally ill people
	• To reduce the overall suicide rate by at least 15%
	• To reduce the suicide rate of severely mentally ill people by at least 33%

The government said that these lives would be saved by five main approaches: earlier diagnosis and treatment of mental illness before it leads to suicide, better targeting of mental health services, better supervision of suicidal people, better support for vulnerable people at stressful times, and less access to methods of suicide (see Box 4).

BOX 4 **Ways the government and NHS can prevent suicide**

- Earlier diagnosis and treatment of mental illness

GPs are being trained and advised on how to recognize depression more easily

- Better targeting of mental health services

People at high risk of suicide should benefit from the NHS's general move to more local and community-based mental health services, as well as from better programmes of care after discharge from hospital

- Better supervision of suicidal people

People known to be suicidal should be supported and supervised very closely, whether in hospital or at home. And patients should always be assessed thoroughly after parasuicide and offered help as appropriate

- Better support during stressful life events

Bereavement counselling, for instance, should be widely available

- Less access to methods of suicide

Since 1992 standards for car exhaust emissions have been tightened and since January 1993 all new cars must have catalytic converters

Warning labels on bottles of poisons, especially

> paracetamol, saying that impulsive overdoses are always potentially fatal
>
> Requiring manufacturers to add to drugs commonly used in overdoses small doses of chemicals that induce vomiting if taken in large quantities or, in the case of paracetamol, to include an antidote in the tablets

---

Earlier recognition and treatment of depression by GPs is crucial, given that half of all suicides result from depression. GPs would be even more effective if they had an anti-suicide pill to prescribe. Many are already prescribing a group of drugs which theoretically fit this bill: the new antidepresants called SSRIs (see p. 76). These are the selective serotonin reuptake inhibitors which increase concentrations of serotonin in the brain. According to the serotonin theory of suicidal behaviour, these drugs should prevent suicide. They are known to relieve and often cure depression, and that is obviously an important indirect way of reducing suicide. But whether SSRIs would prevent suicide in people who intended to kill themselves but were not actually depressed has yet to be confirmed by research.

PARASUICIDE

'Call your mother, Gigi! Liane d'Exelmans has committed suicide.'

The child replied with a long drawn-out 'Oooh!' and asked, 'Is she dead?'

'Of course not. She knows what she's about.'

'How did she do it, Grandmamma? A revolver?'

Madame Alvarez looked pityingly at her granddaughter. 'The idea! Laudanum, as usual. "Doctors Moreze and Pelledoux, who have never left the heart-broken beauty's bedside, cannot yet answer for her life, but their diagnosis is reassuring . . ." My own diagnosis is that if Madame d'Exelmans goes on playing that game, she'll end by ruining her stomach.'

'The last time she killed herself, Grandmamma, was for the sake of Prince Georgevitch, wasn't it?'[3]

Colette's book *Gigi* was first published in 1944, nearly 20 years before the great surge in non-fatal self-harm, or parasuicide, in the developed world. Her light-hearted account may seem flippant, but it reflects a time when the difference between people who intended to kill themselves and those who did not was probably clearer. Since then, the drugs industry's important efforts to make all medicines less toxic may have blurred the distinction. Around 15% of people who harm themselves enough to need medical attention are mentally ill. Some of them may intend to die but fail to do so because the drugs they overdose on are not harmful enough.

Most people who harm themselves non-fatally say that they wanted to blot out and escape from their problems for a while. The decision is usually impulsive, made less than an hour before the act. It is nearly always made alone and in desperation when there seems to be no other way to express distress and attract help. Only a third of people who commit parasuicide say that they really meant to die. It is possible, of course, that some have changed their minds since surviving the act and cannot admit to or cope with having felt really suicidal.

Causes of Parasuicide
As for suicide, annual statistics for parasuicide show certain trends. In most countries statistics on mortality (causes of death) are collected routinely and fairly reliably but those on morbidity (causes of illness and admission to hospital) are not generally collected in the same breadth and depth. Thus, information about national and international trends in parasuicide is less complete than that on suicide.

It seems, however, that certain factors such as social deprivation and unemployment may predispose to both. General similarities and differences between parasuicide and suicide are shown in Box 5.

BOX 5

	SUICIDE	*PARASUICIDE*
Comparing general facts about suicide and parasuicide in the UK		
Cases per year per 100,000 population	10	300
Seasonal variation	spring peak	none
Average age	late 50s	early 20s
Gender	mostly M	mostly F
Commonest social class	upper	lower
Marital status	D>W>S>M*	D & S
Social isolation	yes	maybe
Location	cities	cities
Employment	none/retired	none
Method	violence/OD	mainly OD
Mental illness	90%	15%
Alcohol and drugs	dependent	intoxicated
Life stresses	chronic	acute

For example, the parasuicide rate among unemployed men is 10–15 times higher than that among employed men of the same age. But mental illness is rarer before parasuicide than before suicide. Only 5–8% have serious illness such as schizophrenia or major depression. A further 7–10% have milder

* Suicide is commonest amongst the divorced (D), followed by the widowed (W) and single (S); married (M) people are least likely to commit suicide

depression and anxiety. But up to half of people who harm themselves may have personality disorders, which are discussed in detail in Chapter 7. One subtype, borderline personality disorder, seems to make people particularly impulsive and prone to hurting themselves, often by cutting their wrists superficially and repeatedly.

The most likely candidate for parasuicide is a young woman under acute stress, for example because a close relationship has just ended. She may have chronic stresses too, such as unemployment and an unhappy family life, but she is unlikely to be physically or mentally ill. She will probably take an overdose of common pain-killing tablets such as paracetamol or aspirin, and she may well be drunk at the time. Although alcohol is a contributing factor in successful suicide – a quarter of people who kill themselves have serious alcohol or drug problems and a sixth of all alcoholics eventually commit suicide – it tends to be only a catalyst that intoxicates, reduces inhibitions, and dilutes reason in parasuicide. Nicola, described here, was drunk when she took an overdose:

Nicola was brought into casualty by ambulance at 10 o'clock in the morning. According to the ambulance crew, she had taken an overdose of tablets; probably paracetamol and the sleeping pill temazepam. She had been found unconscious at home half an hour earlier but had roused during the journey to hospital. She was now sleepy but emotional.

A nurse asked Nicola some questions; a doctor asked some more and examined her. The doctor wanted to know what, when, and how much Nicola had taken, and whether she had been sick. She hadn't. After taking some blood for tests, the doctor had to go and see another patient. The nurse returned and explained that Nicola would have to swallow a tube like a small hose to allow her stomach to be washed or 'pumped' out. It sounded terrible, and it proved to be pretty unpleasant.

Nicola felt that she was in some sort of nightmare.

Her head throbbed, she felt sick, and she couldn't stop crying. All she wanted was to see her husband, Geoff. The casualty staff all seemed too busy to spend any time with her. One nurse, though, seemed nice and she promised to ring Geoff at work and ask him to come to the ward where Nicola was going to be admitted.

Nicola was 20. She and Geoff had been married three months. She hadn't been too worried about finding a job straight away; she wanted time to get to know her new town first. And because Geoff's new job as junior manager at the local superstore was quite demanding Nicola wanted to spend some time just being his wife, making sure that he always came home to a good meal and a tidy flat. But it wasn't working out.

Increasingly, Geoff was coming home to a row, mainly about work or money. Geoff's income was enough to cover the mortgage and the bills but there was nothing left for a car, or for a social life, let alone for holidays or other luxuries. He wanted Nicola to look for work.

Nicola had enjoyed her last job as a receptionist and had started some telephonist training. But she seemed to have lost confidence and she kept putting off the decision. Worse than that, she seemed jealous of Geoff's job. He enjoyed it and had already made several friends. They were all single, and whenever Nicola and Geoff met them at the pub they seemed to talk only about women, particularly the women at work.

On the night before Nicola's overdose she had had a huge row with Geoff. They were meant to be going to the store's Christmas party at a big hotel but, at the last minute, Nicola refused to go. She said she felt ill with a bad headache. Geoff didn't believe her and said that she was just being stuck up because she didn't like his friends. Eventually he left, half an hour late, without her.

Initially Nicola was furious. Then she felt miserable, and phoned her mother. It all came out – how she couldn't face finding a job and how she feared that Geoff would lose interest in her. Sobbing, she said she wished she could just have a long sleep and get away from it all for a while. Her mother calmed her down and arranged to visit at the weekend. They would see each other at Christmas, too, and that was only a couple of weeks away.

When Geoff came home at one in the morning he was drunk but amiable. He asked cheerfully about Nicola's headache and went straight to sleep. He overslept and had to rush off to work in the morning, leaving no time to talk. Nicola stayed in bed until 8.30, trying to catch up on some of the sleep that she had missed during what had been a miserable night.

In fact Nicola hadn't slept well for weeks. When she got up that morning she couldn't face the ironing or the cleaning and just sat in front of the television. Hoping that a few drinks might cheer her up, she opened a bottle of vodka. But it didn't help and just made her feel more upset. And now her head did hurt.

Taking a couple of paracetamol tablets for her headache, Nicola suddenly decided to take more. She washed 10 or 11 down with more vodka and, for good measure, took the few sleeping tablets that her mother had given her when she had had trouble sleeping before the wedding.

The next thing Nicola knew of was a loud banging noise. The police were trying to get in the front door. The window cleaner had seen Nicola lying on the floor and had called the police and an ambulance.

On the medical ward where she was eventually sent from casualty Nicola sat between an old lady who seemed unconscious and another who seemed not to be able to breathe properly. A nurse came to ask more questions and take her blood pressure, and then a doctor arrived who explained that Nicola must have a drip in her arm. The amount of paracetamol that Nicola had taken was poisonous and could still kill her unless an antidote was given intravenously. While the drip was being inserted, Geoff arrived with a huge bouquet of flowers.

The following morning two people came to interview Nicola. One, to her horror, was a psychiatrist. The other was a social worker. They asked detailed questions about her life, her worries, and the events of the previous day. To Nicola's relief, they seemed to understand what had been happening to her.

Preventing Parasuicide

What People Who Feel Suicidal Can Do
A sympathetic ear is the first port of call for people who want to overcome urges to harm themselves. Those who cannot bear to tell a relative, a friend, or a professional like a GP can phone the Samaritans. The address of their national office is given in the directory at the back of this book. Local branches are listed in telephone directories and guides to local services. Whatever the time of day, the Samaritans will answer and listen. Callers don't have to say who they are. Talking things through can help to make sense of feelings and reduce the suicidal impulse. Specialized counselling services and 24-hour helplines, for instance for alcohol and drug problems or young people's problems, can also help.

It is often possible to do something positive to reduce suicidal feelings. Lonely people and those with problems at home may be able to go and stay somewhere safe, perhaps with friends or family. And they can make sure that they keep busy, preferably by doing something that is potentially enjoyable rather than stressful, until the feelings pass. People who feel they might harm themselves impulsively can remove all dangerous objects and substances (especially painkillers and alcohol) from the house. And those who feel anger can try to direct it at the right source, perhaps by having a huge row with the person who is causing the feelings.

What Friends and Relatives Can Do

It is sometimes very difficult to imagine how people are feeling if they do not tell you. But research has shown that one emotion in particular, hopelessness, is intrinsic to most suicide. If someone ill or under stress starts saying deeply pessimistic things like 'I have no future' or 'I've lost everything', relatives and friends should try to get him or her to talk about the feeling in more detail. Even if the person isn't usually communicative, he or she may become so before suicide. For instance, up to 15% of people with schizophrenia eventually kill themselves and they most commonly do it when they are lucid, not psychotic, and have realized the severity of their illness. And there is a myth that people who threaten suicide do not really mean it. In fact, up to two-thirds of people who die by suicide tell someone of their intentions just beforehand.

Relatives and friends should take such warnings seriously and listen. Listening sympathetically to a suicidal person's fears and feelings can prevent disaster. But this may leave listeners so alarmed and confused, and so unsure whether they can deal with this alone, that they should persuade the person to get some professional help.

Even if the person accepts professional help, support from relatives and friends may be needed for some time. If the suicidal person lives with them, they may be tempted to take over and start trying to control him or her. This is often counterproductive. It is better to discuss things openly and to treat a suicidal person as a generally responsible adult. The person can be watched closely and any obvious means of self-harm can be removed from the house without being too heavy-handed. Overprotectiveness, even in such a crisis, often makes suicidal people feel more worthless.

If someone repeatedly threatens suicide but does not accept or respond to help, those close to them may find it increasingly difficult to sympathize. They may find it hard, too, to believe in the psychiatrists or other professionals involved because they seem so ineffectual. But it is worth working at a relationship with the professionals because they are often able to support relatives and friends. And perhaps one or other side of this relationship will notice a change in the nature of the suicidal person's repeated threats. This is important and is worth discussing because it may signal real intent to die. Some people who repeatedly threaten suicide do eventually kill themselves.

What Professionals Can Do

Parasuicide causes great personal harm and suffering and costs the NHS a lot of money. These are all good reasons to prevent it, but even more importantly, preventing parasuicide indirectly reduces suicide. People who commit parasuicide are 100 times more likely than the general population to kill themselves in the next year.

Public services like the NHS and social services have clear roles and policies for trying to prevent parasuicide and suicide. The NHS has three main responsibilities towards parasuicidal patients: emergency treatment, thorough assessment of suicide risk, and treatment for any related physical or mental illness. Social services departments have responsibilities towards people with social problems.

The idea that people who harm themselves need care and support is fairly recent in Britain. After all, deliberate self-harm was illegal from 1554 to 1961. Then, through the 1961 Suicide Act, the Ministry of Health acknowledged the importance of checking thoroughly for suicide risk after parasuicide and recommended that all parasuicidal patients should be seen by psychiatrists. Later advice was that all should be admitted to general hospitals for observation.

In 1984, however, the Department of Health and Social Security drew up the current guidelines suggesting that any doctor (such as a casualty officer or GP) or a non-doctor with special training (such as a social worker) could make the assessment and decide whether to refer on to a psychiatrist. These guidelines imply that not all such patients need be admitted to hospital if there is no further risk to life. This could apply to people who impulsively take a few non-lethal tablets or superficially cut themselves in response to straightforward, transient triggers like arguments. One study showed that nearly a fifth of patients who poison themselves and go to casualty are discharged after assessment and appropriate treatment without being admitted to the hospital.[4] For most patients, assessment and treatment will include the following:

EMERGENCY ASSESSMENT AND TREATMENT
A doctor will examine the patient and will need to know as much as possible about the damage inflicted. Cuts, bruises, and other injuries should be self-explanatory but patients may have to give details if they have poisoned themselves. What tablets did they take? When? How many? Other information can be obtained from tests, particularly blood tests to see the level of poison in the body and the degree of harm done.

Then the doctor may have to give treatment, and it is often unpleasant. Cuts may need stitching and fractures setting. Poison may have to be flushed out of the system by pouring salty water down the throat (to wash or 'pump' out the stomach) or using medicines such as emetics (to cause vomiting), charcoal tablets (to mop up the poison from the intestine), and drugs to encourage the elimination of the poison in the urine. Some poisons need neutralizing by antidotes, usually given by drip into the bloodstream.

Patients may be admitted to a general medical ward for at least a night, particularly if they are very sleepy, if they have hurt themselves badly, or the required treatment is complicated and lengthy. Some may need surgery. The next of kin will be contacted and patients will, of course, be allowed to have visitors.

FURTHER ASSESSMENT
Before being assessed fully, patients should be given time to recover from the effects of the overdose or other self-harm. It is unfair and often uninformative to interview someone who is still drowsy from sedatives or still upset from repair of cut wrists.

People seen first by their GP and judged not to be in need

of referral to hospital for emergency treatment may not need to be interviewed by anyone else. Those who go to hospital are usually interviewed by one or more members of a psychiatric team – a psychiatrist, a social worker, or a psychiatric nurse. They will see patients in private if possible; in a side room rather than the open ward. They will need to know what led up to the self-harm and what has been happening in patients' lives (see Box 6). They may also take a brief psychiatric history (see pp. xvii–xxi).

BOX 6

Questions asked during assessment after parasuicide

a. About the act:

- How did you spend the day before harming yourself?

- Where, when, and how did you harm yourself?

- What did you think would happen to you afterwards? (Did you realize the danger?)

- Did you intend to kill yourself?

- If not, what did you intend?

- Did you tell anyone or leave a note?

- Did you expect to be found?

- Do you think you will harm yourself again?

b. About your problems:

- Have you any problems?

- How are you going to sort them out?

- Have you family and friends who could help you?

- Do you need professional help?

c. About your health:

- Have you harmed yourself before?

- Have you felt ill (physically or mentally) recently or in the past?
- If so, have you had any help or treatment?

These interviews often help patients. They provide a chance to talk about feelings and about what happened. For the professionals it is a chance to see whether patients really meant to kill themselves and whether they need further help. Bearing in mind the known risks for suicide, and perhaps using special questionnaires (which suggest increased risk if people score highly on certain questions), they will try to assess the likelihood of patients repeating the act and killing themselves next time.

The professionals sometimes find evidence of mental illness or personality disorder and refer patients for further psychiatric help. If illness is bad enough to need treatment with drugs, the risk of overdosing on them must be taken into account. Relatives or friends may be asked to keep the medicines safe.

Admission to a psychiatric hospital may be necessary, and patients who refuse to go but are considered a continuing risk to themselves may be legally forced to go. Compulsory psychiatric admission (certifying or sectioning) under a section of the Mental Health Act is only used in extreme circumstances and patients have the right to appeal against it. The procedures used and rights protected under the Act are explained in detail in Chapter 9.

Some kind of follow up may be recommended even for people who are not ill. About one-third of parasuicide patients benefit from a few sessions of counselling, often given at a psychiatric outpatient clinic. Counselling and advice on social problems may be offered by the local social services department.

Outcome of Treatment for Parasuicide
Many parasuicide patients find that the worried and helpful responses by their families, friends, and the professionals are

enough to solve their problems. This is how Nicola, whose story was described above, felt:

Geoff had mistaken Nicola's lack of confidence for jealousy and had not noticed how miserable she had become. In hospital they talked and talked and resolved that they would work hard at settling into the new town together. Geoff would help Nicola to get to know his workmates more gradually and they would both join the local sports club to make new friends jointly. Nicola agreed to try the job that a family friend had offered. At least she would know someone there. When she woke the next morning in hospital she felt much better; almost back to her old self.

Nicola was surprised, therefore, when the psychiatrist and social worker suggested that she needed some counselling. They wanted to check that her improvement would last because there were a few aspects of her story that worried them. Firstly, her general unhappiness, her insomnia, and the fact that she took the overdose in the morning suggested that she might have been becoming depressed. Most people who impulsively commit parasuicide do it in the evening, often after a disastrous evening out with too much alcohol. People with depression feel at their lowest in the morning. Thus, the psychiatrist offered to see Nicola in the outpatient clinic.

For a very small minority the attention gained after parasuicide is so gratifying that they try self-harm again. The risks are high, though. For a start, there is the physical risk and secondly, there is the considerable risk that the people whose attention is wanted will lose patience and eventually lose interest. Other people try again because they still feel bad. In all, about one in ten of parasuicide patients eventually kill themselves.

Suicide is devastating for the families and friends left behind. Professional help sometimes helps them to cope.

Help for Relatives and Friends after Suicide

It can take years to feel normal after any bereavement. But suicide is particularly painful. Those left may feel guilty that they couldn't prevent it. They may be angry with the person who died, and feel guilty about that. And they may be angry with the doctors and other professionals who knew the person but didn't prevent the suicide.

Many relatives find the distress of a public inquest particularly hard to cope with. All deaths that are sudden, violent, or unexpected; due to injury, accident, or poisoning; or of unknown or suspicious cause must be reported to a coroner. The coroner will discuss the cause of death with the doctor of the deceased and may request a postmortem and a police inquiry. Whatever the outcome of these investigations, the coroner has to order an inquest when the death is not clearly due to natural causes. Only when a verdict is reached can the coroner issue a death certificate and thereby allow the funeral to take place. A verdict of suicide can be used only when there is proof that the deceased intended to take his or her own life. Otherwise, an open verdict must be given. The police officers, coroners, and journalists involved (the verdict is often reported in the local newspaper) will usually handle the inquest as sensitively as possible, but relatives may find that the investigations and delays are the last straw.

Grief usually declines after about a year. If it does not, or if the bereaved person still experiences some of the symptoms of grief that are common (and normal) in the first few months, such as hearing the dead person's voice or seeing them transiently, they may need special help (see pp. 61–3). GPs can refer patients for bereavement counselling. And the national organization for bereaved people, CRUSE, which has many local branches, can provide counselling and support.

9 ETHICAL AND LEGAL ASPECTS OF PSYCHIATRY

The Psychiatrist's Dilemma

> If a madman were to come into this room with a stick in his hand, no doubt we should pity the state of his mind; but our primary consideration would be to take care of ourselves. We should knock him down first, and pity him afterwards.
>
> From *The Life of Samuel Johnson* by James Boswell

> What the public wants is a cheap magic charm to prevent, and a cheap pill or potion to cure, all disease. It forces all such charms on the doctors.
>
> From *The Doctor's Dilemma* by George Bernard Shaw[1]

In George Bernard Shaw's preface to his play *The Doctor's Dilemma* he described doctoring as an art, practised by men no more scientific than their tailors. He spared them little sympathy when they tried to use ignorance as defence against malpractice, pointing out that doctors themselves claimed to know everything and enjoyed their power. Even today, both society and the medical profession seem to expect unrealistically perfect practice and give doctors a great deal of influence. Psychiatrists have a special power and a special dilemma; they can shut people away.

When a person is too ill to give or even withhold consent but psychiatric help is considered essential, the law allows that help to be given anyway – within strict guidelines. Often there is no doubt in the minds of the family and the health care workers involved that such a course of action is necessary because all else has failed. However, there are times when the professionals are asked to take away an individual's freedom for reasons that are perhaps more social than medical. For example, a person may be causing an unexplained disturbance in the street. Local residents, alarmed and annoyed, may insist that something should be done and demand that the person is taken to hospital. The person may be showing outward signs which strongly suggest mental illness, but may not feel unwell or consider his behaviour to be unusual. The police may call in a doctor and a social worker, who recommend and arrange admission to a psychiatric hospital for assessment. In this situation a person can be deprived of freedom by certain health care workers acting as a kind of social police force.

The stereotyped example of this is of a violent, disturbed person who is arrested and sent to hospital after assaulting an innocent bystander. But many people who are sent to psychiatric hospitals against their will are simply ill; so ill that they cannot understand the need for treatment. Sarah's story is much more typical than the lurid stereotype:

Sarah was 58 and married, with three grown up children. She had always thought of herself as a bit of a worrier and had felt low after the birth of her youngest child, but had never sought any help for her 'nerves'. Her husband John was 64 and planning retirement from his job as an engineer. Sarah began to worry that they would not be able to maintain a reasonable standard of living, despite the fact that John had a very good pension and had also made other savings and investments. She felt guilty that she had not worked and contributed to the household budget over the years. John tried to reassure her, but she became completely preoccupied with these worries and within a month she had lost her appetite and half a stone in weight. She woke early in the mornings, feeling so desperate that she could barely face the coming day.

One night Sarah woke with a start at 3 a.m. and walked out of the house in her nightclothes. She was muddled and agitated, saying that John would be much better off without her. He had been woken by the front door banging and he managed to calm her enough to take her back into the house.

John called his family doctor, who talked with Sarah. Although she denied any ideas of harming herself, she could not be swayed from her irrational ideas that she and John were on the verge of financial ruin because of her idleness in not having a job outside the home. She even told her doctor to call the police so that she could be taken to prison for some unspecific crime.

The GP said that Sarah was very depressed, needing urgent psychiatric help. He felt that she was potentially suicidal and it also worried him that she had barely eaten for a week. It might be possible for her to be seen in a psychiatric outpatient clinic in the next day or two, or be visited at home by a specialist. Sarah refused to see a psychiatrist, protesting that she was 'bad, not mad'.

The doctor decided that there would be little hope of persuading Sarah to accept any help at home, so he recommended a stay in hospital. She refused this too, despite reassurance from John. The doctor called in a social worker and a senior psychiatrist who were both on night duty for emergencies. After talking with Sarah and then with John, the two doctors and the social worker signed special application forms to admit Sarah to the local psychiatric hospital for assessment and help.

All these arrangements took time but by the morning Sarah had arrived in the admission ward. John and the social worker had taken her there by car, and although she still maintained that it was a waste of time she did not try to resist at all. Once she had met the staff and some of the other patients, Sarah seemed resigned and went off to look round the ward. John went home once she had settled in a little. He felt a mixture of worry and relief; he could not have coped any longer with her at home in that state.

This kind of emergency happens several times a week in every town. Is it right that an individual can be admitted to hospital against his or her will? Should doctors and social workers have this much power? In Common Law people's affairs can be handed over to other appointed individuals only after the courts have agreed that they cannot manage them. Mental health law, however, gives responsibility for two personal affairs – liberty and self-care – to certain professionals without going through the courts. A label of probable mental illness is all that is needed. This threatens individual freedom. But in the long term mental illness can do far greater damage to personal liberty. In our society treatment of illness has become a basic right; thus failure to be treated when mentally ill ignores that right and discriminates against a vulnerable group. Surely people with mental problems are as entitled to treatment as those with physical illness.

Doctors, therefore, have to balance the rights of patients against their own duties to provide treatment. Doctors in the United Kingdom have a duty to follow certain standards of practice as laid down by the General Medical Council. This controlling body, established in 1858, produces a register of all qualified doctors from which a practitioner's name may be struck off if found guilty of misconduct. One of the most important requirements is that a registered medical practitioner will 'afford and maintain a good standard of medical care'. This includes 'appropriate and prompt action upon existence of a condition requiring urgent medical intervention'. A doctor who fails to provide or arrange treatment for a patient when necessary may be disciplined.

To take away a person's freedom and treat him against his will could be a serious infringement of civil rights. And other restrictions on the lives of certain patients in psychiatric hospitals, which affect things like sending and receiving correspondence and voting in political elections, could be equally serious. The law maker's and psychiatrist's dilemma is knowing how to respect general civil rights without depriving patients of a specific right, namely, health care.

MENTAL HEALTH LAW

Early legislation for people with mental problems in England dealt only with the management of any property they might own. The law referred to 'lunatics or persons of unsound mind', who were thought likely to recover, and 'natural fools or idiots' who were considered incurable. There were a few public institutions for these people but many ended up in gaols, poorhouses and workhouses. Physical restraint was the only treatment available for most people.

The 18th century saw the first law which allowed the arrest and detention of 'potentially dangerous persons' on the order of two judges. Later Acts of Parliament said that no person should be detained in this way unless he or she was behaving very abnormally. Certain standards of care for detained persons were expected by law.

In the 19th century people with mental health problems were considered on a large scale for the first time. Over 20 Acts ordered special accommodation for 'idiots, imbeciles and lunatics'. These institutions were called county asylums, aiming to live up to the literal meaning of the word asylum as a place of refuge and sanctuary.

The 1930 Mental Treatment Act replaced the terms 'lunatic' and 'asylum' with 'person of unsound mind' and 'mental hospital', because the old words had attracted social stigma. The Act also provided for voluntary admission, not generally possible before. By the late 1950s admission to a psychiatric hospital in the early stages of illness was encouraged because advances in treatment were producing good results. Physical treatments included electroconvulsive therapy (ECT), effective antipsychotic and antidepressant drugs, and psychosurgery. Psychoanalysis was also increasingly available and attractive.

By 1957 three-quarters of all admissions were voluntary. The 1959 Mental Health Act allowed psychiatric hospitals to provide better care for the majority of their clientele, i.e. patients who had agreed to be there. Doors were unlocked and health authorities began to provide outpatient clinics. Compulsory care was only allowed within quite strict limits and certain time periods. Patients could be detained by legal restraint rather than physical in most cases. Patients knew that they had to stay in hospital and that they could be brought back if they tried to leave during a certain period of time. This was usually enough to prevent them from trying to go, and ward doors did not have to be locked.

In 1983 the Mental Health Act for England and Wales was amended on the recommendations of a special Royal Commission and the mental health charity MIND. Most of the changes reduced the extent of the law, making overuse of emergency powers less likely and increasing the rights of patients to appeal against being detained. It is this Act of 1983 that is used currently in England and Wales. In 1989 the Act applied to about 5% of all patients in psychiatric hospitals; thus more than nine out of 10 were admitted voluntarily.

Scotland's legal system is different from that in England and Wales. Therefore its mental health laws are different, governed by the Mental Health (Scotland) Act 1984. The basic intentions and powers of the Scottish Act are broadly the same, however. So are those of the Mental Health (Northern Ireland) Order 1986.

Current Mental Health Legislation:
The Mental Health Act 1983

This Act is mainly used to authorize the admission to psychiatric hospital of a person who seems to need it but has refused it. Different parts or sections of the Act deal with different parts of this process. Rather than using long-winded phrases like 'compulsory admission under Section 2 of the Mental Health Act 1983' the noun 'section' has been developed into a verb in practical usage. For example, a relative may be told 'I'm afraid we'll have to section him if he refuses to come to hospital.' (The words 'certify' and 'commit' were once used in the same way.) A section may also be called an order. A person who is admitted or treated under a section is called a compulsory or formal patient. A person who has agreed to either kind of help and is not on a section is called a voluntary or informal patient.

Like any piece of legislation the Mental Health Act is complicated and full of jargon. The basic powers and rights it confers are summarized in Box 1.

BOX 1

Mental Health Act 1983 – Basic Powers and Rights
Minimum Loss of Liberty The Act states clearly that the least restrictive course of effective action should be taken at all times. Thus a person should be sectioned only when all other possibilities are exhausted or inappropriate. Compulsory admission does not automatically or usually lead to restraint or locked doors. *Patients' Rights* Anyone sectioned must have their rights explained, including those of appeal. All sections or orders of more than 72 hours' duration confer rights of appeal. *Relatives' Rights and Powers* The Act gives sectioned patients' nearest relatives important powers – it does not give power only to professionals.

The Framework of the Act

PEOPLE COVERED BY THE ACT

The Mental Health Act can be used for anyone who has a mental disorder which is threatening their own health or safety, or that of others, and is refusing psychiatric help. The

Act calls such a person the patient, whether or not in hospital. In psychiatric slang someone who is sufficiently ill or handicapped to be sectioned may be described as sectionable.

Someone who is apparently mentally disordered but is coping adequately with life and is not harming anyone else should not be sectioned. After all, being strange is not a crime: people should have the right to be strange if they like. But the Act is not meant to be so narrow that it is reserved only for the severely mentally ill who are in danger of harming themselves or others. It can be used in the interests of someone's health, not only their safety. This clause is important, but it seems to have been misinterpreted many times in the past, as if it said 'health and safety' rather than 'health or safety'. Relatives often say that they have to watch someone getting more and more ill before the professionals, who may be erring on the side of caution for fear of transgressing civil rights, decide to use the Act.

Decisions about whether someone is risking health and safety are, of course, subjective. And so is the definition of mental disorder. Mental health problems do not always fit easily into categories with specific labels. The Mental Health Act gets round this by avoiding detailed definitions of mental disorder. It defines mental disorder broadly as 'mental illness, arrested or incomplete development of mind, psychopathic disorder and any other disorder or disability of mind'. Mental disorder is then subdivided into four separate groups: mental illness, mental impairment, severe mental impairment and psychopathic disorder.

PROBLEMS COVERED BY THE ACT
Mental illness This is not defined any further, creating a seemingly gaping hole in the Act. Presumably any attempt at definition could have been too narrow or too easy to abuse. In 1973 Lord Justice Lawton said that because the Act used ordinary words of the English language, rather than technical jargon, the law should define mental illness as any ordinary sensible person would do. He confirmed, therefore, some people's view that mental illness is defined by society.

Mental impairment This is defined as 'a state of arrested or incomplete development of mind which includes significant impairment of intelligence and social functioning and is associated with abnormally aggressive or seriously irresponsible conduct on the part of the person concerned'. Instead of the term 'impairment' the 1959 Act used 'subnormality', which was dropped because it suggested that such people were substandard people. The intention was to replace it with handicap in the new Act. However, a number of organizations, most notably the charity for mentally handicapped children and adults (MENCAP), protested at the inclusion of handicapped people in the Act at all. They argued that care, rather than treatment, was needed for people with these problems and that it could nearly always be provided outside hospitals.

Despite this valid point it was felt that a very small proportion of mentally handicapped people might need compulsory psychiatric help if they were behaving in ways which posed risks to themselves or others. The Act uses the term impairment to sidestep this argument. And, because the word handicap has itself attracted stigma, people with such problems are now called (except in the Mental Health Act) people with learning disabilities.

Severe mental impairment is defined in the same way except that the word significant is replaced by severe.

Psychopathic disorder This is a type of personality disorder. Personality disorder is the psychiatric name for a long-term problem of social behaviour, attitudes and emotions. Psychopathic personality disorder is the name for a problem of persistently antisocial behaviour and little concern for other people: a sort of grown-up delinquency. These labels are morally and socially tricky concepts that are discussed in much more detail in Chapter 7.

The Mental Health Act defines psychopathic disorder as 'a persistent disorder or disability of mind (whether or not including significant impairment of intelligence) which results in abnormally aggressive or seriously irresponsible conduct on the part of the person concerned'.

WHO USES THE ACT

Any doctor can use certain sections of the Mental Health Act. But those with the widest powers are senior psychiatrists who the Act refers to as approved doctors and responsible medical officers. An approved doctor is one with higher qualifications in psychiatry who has been recognized by the Secretary of State for Health as having special experience in diagnosing or treating mental disorder. A responsible medical officer (RMO) is a senior psychiatrist (usually a consultant) in charge of the overall care of a sectioned patient. GPs are the other group of doctors most closely involved in deciding whether patients should be sectioned. Several sections require the opinions of two doctors, one of whom has known the patient for some time if possible. This is nearly always the GP.

Social workers and patients' relatives can use certain sections of the Act in conjunction with doctors. Social workers have to have sufficient qualifications and special training in mental health and the law before they can call themselves approved social workers (ASWs) and use the Act. Patients' nearest relatives, as defined by the Act (see Box 2) can, within certain limits, apply for compulsory admission, appeal against a section, and order discharge of a relative who is considered mentally disordered. The relative must also be informed of any actions under the Act which affect that person. In the past all relatives had powers under mental health law but this proved to be too wide a range for the best interests of the patient.

BOX 2	**Nearest relatives as defined by the Mental Health Act**
	a. spouse (if the couple are not permanently separated)
	b. child
	c. parent
	d. brother or sister
	e. grandparent

f. grandchild

g. uncle or aunt

h. nephew or niece

The elder parent takes precedence over the younger. A relative with whom the patient usually lives takes priority over others, as does anyone (even if unrelated) with whom he or she has lived for more than five years.

Finally, hospital managers (administrators) play a part on behalf of the local health authority. They provide and file the legal forms that doctors, social workers, and relatives fill in when using the Mental Health Act. They also oversee the day to day use of the Act, reminding staff of expiry dates of sections and organizing tribunals (see below).

The overall use of the Mental Health Act throughout England and Wales is monitored by a government-appointed body called the Mental Health Act Commission. The commission recruits members who may be psychiatrists, psychologists, nurses, social workers, lawyers or lay people who work for the commission for up to four years. Members visit patients on sections, investigate their complaints, and lay down rules or codes of practice that govern general ethics and the use of the Act. They also provide independent expert advice to social workers and doctors, including second opinions before certain treatments can be given against patients' wishes. In Scotland the law is supervised by the Mental Welfare Commission; Northern Ireland has its own Mental Health Commission.

Undoing a Section

Most sections of the 1983 Act can order patients to stay in hospital or to take treatment only for certain lengths of time. The orders or sections then expire, although they can be continued if further legal steps are taken. Sections do not have to run until the expiry date, however. If detained patients recover enough to accept care and treatment voluntarily, their sections can be undone before expiry. Responsible medical officers and hospital managers have the power to undo sections and discharge patients from compulsory care and treatment. Discharge from a section does not necessarily equate with discharge from hospital, however: it simply means that the patient is now able to comply with the recommended programme of care.

Nearest relatives can also order discharge from some sections by writing to the hospital managers. Unless the responsible medical officer makes a report stating that the patient must stay in hospital, discharge has to be granted within three days of the request.

APPEALING AGAINST A SECTION

Patients who are subject to the 1984 Act in Scotland can appeal to the Mental Welfare Commission or to a Sheriff. In England and Wales patients can appeal to independent bodies called Mental Health Review Tribunals which hear the cases for and against individual sections. Tribunal members are appointed by the Lord Chancellor, the chief judge in the United Kingdom. In each area of the country there is a tribunal chairman, a lawyer, who is responsible for organizing panels including lay people with knowledge of social services or related topics, experienced lawyers, and senior psychiatrists who are not connected with the local hospitals.

A patient or, in certain circumstances, a nearest relative can appeal to a tribunal hearing by filling in an application form obtained from the hospital. This form must be sent to the local Mental Health Review Tribunal office within a certain time. Every patient who is held on a section is given written details of this procedure as part of the admission routine. A patient who has been detained for six months without applying to a tribunal will be seen by one automatically.

Once the application has been received a date is arranged for a tribunal hearing, to be held at the hospital where the patient is staying. The independent psychiatrist will come and see the patient in private before the hearing and make a medical assessment. When a patient appeals against compulsory treatment and not just detention, the tribunal has to satisfy itself that the prescribed treatment is likely to improve the patient's quality of life, either by alleviating symptoms or preventing deterioration.

The patient has the right to ask his own representative to attend the hearing, and may choose another lawyer. If the patient does not choose his own lawyer the health authority or the charity MIND (the National Association for Mental Health) will provide one on request. The representative can visit the patient before the hearing and help to prepare for the tribunal. Representatives can involve relatives if asked, arrange second opinions from independent doctors and social workers, and help to find accommodation if discharge is ordered by the tribunal. A limited form of legal aid called assistance by way of representation will pay for all this if the patient cannot afford it.

Tribunals exist to help patients. But they can, unfortunately, seem rather intimidating. They are usually held in a grand committee room in the hospital where the panel sits behind an imposing table. The president of the tribunal (the lawyer) chairs the meeting, letting the patient speak and inviting each panel member to ask the patient about his or her current problems. The responsible medical officer has to explain, in writing and usually in person, why he or she is not recommending early discharge. After everyone has spoken the patient is asked to leave the room while the tribunal decides what to do. This may take an hour or more, particularly if there are other hearings taking place that day.

The tribunal will order discharge if it does not find the patient to be suffering from mental disorder or if detention cannot be justified in the interests of the patient's health and safety or that of others. It may recommend discharge in a few days' time so that the patient does not rush out of hospital without making any plans for accommodation or allowing the psychiatric team to plan and offer continuing help.

Sections of the 1983 Act

The Mental Health Act authorizes three main outcomes: compulsory admission for assessment, compulsory treatment, and admission and transfer of people involved in criminal proceedings. The most commonly used parts of the Act are sections 2 and 3. Rather than discussing the sections in order of use, however, it is probably clearer to discuss them in order of duration, starting with the shortest. These are summarized in Box 3. For consistency with the Act the term 'patient' and the pronoun 'he' is used throughout this discussion.

BOX 3

> **Summary of the Mental Health Act 1983, England and Wales**
>
> Detention for up to 72 hours
>
> Sections 4, 136, 135, 5
>
> Detention for up to 28 days
>
> Sections 2, 35, 36
>
> Detention for six months or longer
>
> Sections 3, 37, 47, 41
>
> Guardianship for six months or longer
>
> Section 7
>
> Consent to treatment
>
> Sections 57, 58, 62

DETENTION FOR UP TO 72 HOURS

Section 4: Admission for assessment in emergencies   This should be used only when it is 'of urgent necessity' for the patient to be admitted to hospital and kept there because he appears to be suffering from a mental disorder which threatens his own health or safety or that of others. An approved social worker or the patient's nearest relative signs an application form and calls any doctor, not necessarily an approved one (see p. 267). Usually the patient's GP is called. If, after seeing the patient, the doctor agrees with the person who has made the application and fills out another form, stating the circumstances of the emergency, he can arrange the admission immediately.

Once in hospital, the patient will not be able to leave before the 72-hour limit expires and will not have any right to appeal. He can refuse treatment. After 72 hours he must be discharged unless he agrees to stay voluntarily or is seen by a psychiatrist who sets up detention under a longer-lasting section.

Ideally, local hospital services should be able to provide a specially approved psychiatrist in any emergency, day or night, so that section 4 is rarely necessary. In most areas of the United Kingdom local psychiatric consultants have duty rotas to cover this and will come to the patient's home.

Section 136: Detention by the police in a place of safety   If someone appears to be mentally disordered in a public place and in immediate need of 'care or control', a police officer can take him to a place of safety and arrange for him to be kept there for up to 72 hours. This place is usually a police station or hospital. No application form or medical opinion is required at first but the purpose of this section is for subsequent examination by a doctor and social worker once the person has been detained. In practice these assessments are more likely to occur quickly at a police station and the psychiatrist called will be a senior one (usually the consultant on call).

Being taken straight to a hospital may seem better than being held in a police cell. But going straight to hospital under section 136 may lead to assessment by a junior psychiatrist (the hospital's duty doctor) who will often have to keep the patient in overnight or over the weekend for assessment by a consultant psychiatrist and social worker on the next working day. This is because someone who is already in a safe place under specialist supervision may be less of a priority for urgent assessment by the duty consultant and social worker than other people outside hospital.

Section 135: Warrant to search and remove patients   This section is used very rarely. It allows a magistrate to issue a warrant which authorizes a police officer, accompanied by a doctor and an approved social worker, to enter any premises and remove a person to a place of safety. There must be reasonable cause to believe that the person is suffering from mental disorder and has been ill treated, neglected, or not kept under proper control; or is living alone and is not capable of caring for himself.

The patient can then be detained in a place of safety (see section 136) but the Department of Health recommends that a police station is used only when immediate admission to hospital is not possible.

Incidentally, there is another law that allows, via a magistrate, 'removal to suitable premises of persons in need of care and attention who are suffering from grave chronic diseases or, being aged, infirm or physically incapacitated, are living in insanitary conditions and are unable to devote to themselves, and are not receiving from other persons, proper care and attention'. This law has nothing to do with the Mental Health Act; it is called the National Assistance Act (1948), section 47. It is used occasionally, for example to take to hospital a hypothermic elderly person who refuses help.

Section 5: Detention of patients who are already in hospital Sometimes patients who are not on sections decide to leave hospital against medical advice. If such a patient is still ill, but able to cope outside hospital without harming himself or anyone else, staff may try to persuade him to stay. If he insists on going, he will usually be asked to sign a form stating that the hospital is no longer responsible for him.

If, however, detention seems necessary, a psychiatric nurse can sign an application form to prevent the patient leaving in the next six hours, until he has been seen by a doctor. This is section 5(4), sometimes called the nurses' holding power.

Doctors (usually the junior ward doctors) can use section 5(2) in the same circumstances to detain a patient for up to 72 hours so that an approved psychiatrist and social worker can be called to assess whether a longer section is needed.

DETENTION FOR UP TO 28 DAYS

Section 2: Admission for assessment   If a person seems to need compulsory admission to hospital and there is enough time to organize visits by two doctors and a social worker, section 2 should be used. The nearest relative, or an approved social worker who has seen the person in the past 14 days, makes an application by stating on a special form that the person is suffering from mental disorder and should be detained in the interests of his own health or safety or that of others.

Two doctors must then see the person. If they do this separately the two examinations must not be more than five days apart. One of the doctors must be an approved psychiatrist; the other, if possible, should know the patient already. The second doctor is usually the patient's GP but if he or she is on holiday or not available another GP can do the assessment.

If the doctors agree with the application they can arrange admission to hospital for up to 28 days. A patient detained under section 2 can be given treatment, even if he does not want it (see p. 280 for more on consent to treatment).

A month is a long time to be forced to stay somewhere and the law recognizes this. On admission to hospital the patient is given an explanation of his rights, including that of appeal. Within the first 14 days of detention he can ask for a tribunal so that he can appeal against being in hospital. The 72-hour sections do not give this chance simply because there would not be time to arrange a tribunal in three days. Under section 2 the patient must be discharged from hospital on the 28th day unless he has decided to stay voluntarily, which is often the case.

In Northern Ireland most initial compulsory assessments last up to seven days, renewable for a further week. There is no equivalent to this in England and Wales.

Sections 35 and 36: Assessment of offenders   Some people who have been charged with criminal offences but have not yet been sentenced are sent to prison on remand. In 1988 just under a quarter of the whole prison population in England and Wales were unsentenced remand prisoners. Remand prisoners have high rates of mental health problems and suicide and many should be in hospital, not prison, if figures on sentenced prisoners are anything to go by.

More than a third of men serving sentences in English and Welsh prisons who were surveyed in 1988 had some kind of mental health problem.[2] The researchers interviewed 5% of all sentenced prisoners nationally, making sure that the men seen represented the total in terms of length of sentence and type of prison. A fifth had alcohol and drug problems. About 2% (equal to around 700 men throughout English and Welsh prisons) had psychotic mental illnesses like schizophrenia. In all, around 1100 men or 3% nationally were considered to need transfer for treatment in psychiatric hospitals.

Yet many prisoners never get to see psychiatrists and those who do while on remand have often been in hospital many months before assessment. In 1992 the Government published the Reed report on services for offenders with mental disorder,[3] drawn up by a committee of experts chaired by Dr John Reed, a senior government doctor. The report recommended that, whenever possible, people who commit crimes while mentally ill should be cared for and treated in hospitals and should not go to prison. Although special laws and services already existed for these offenders, the report said that practice too often fell short of what was desirable. Schemes in which psychiatrists attend court and immediately assess people who seem mentally ill, should be expanded, said the report. Accused but unsentenced offenders who need further assessment or treatment in hospital can be admitted under sections 35, 36, and 38 of the Mental Health Act.

Section 35 allows a remand for assessment for up to 28 days, renewable for two further 28-day periods if necessary. If the person ends up in prison the time spent on remand in hospital will be deducted from the sentence. Section 36 allows a remand to hospital for compulsory treatment for up to 28 days, within the same conditions as section 35. It cannot be used for someone accused of murder. Section 38 authorizes admission to hospital to try compulsory treatment for up to 12 weeks and is renewable.

DETENTION FOR SIX MONTHS OR LONGER

Section 3: Admission for treatment In practice, treatment orders under section 3 are used for patients who have already been diagnosed as mentally ill and are well known to the local psychiatric team. The procedure for admission is the same as that for section 2 but the doctors must be able to say which kind of mental disorder is affecting the patient (mental illness, psychopathic disorder, severe mental impairment, or mental impairment). They must also state that treatment cannot be provided unless the patient is in hospital, usually because the patient would not cooperate with treatment as an outpatient.

When social workers make applications for section 3 they must satisfy themselves that there is no viable alternative to admission. They must also inform the patients' nearest relatives. If a nearest relative disagrees with the planned admission it cannot go ahead unless the objection is overruled by a county court.

Section 3 is also used to keep patients in hospital who have come in voluntarily or on shorter sections but need help for longer. The same procedures are used. This section can be renewed for a further six months and then for periods of one year; the patient can appeal to a tribunal after each renewal.

Some people with long-term mental health problems, particularly schizophrenia, get to a point when they are well enough to leave hospital but still need to keep up with drug treatment and other aspects of care to have the best chance of staying well. Their ability to cope outside hospital will usually have been tested during periods of leave, for instance weekends spent at home. Those on section 3 can be sent out for extended leave under section 17 for up to a year. This allows for compulsory treatment in the community and for compulsory return to hospital if the patient relapses during leave. But in 1986 a leading judge ruled that the Mental Health Act of 1983 would have included a clearly separate order for treating people outside hospital against their will – a community treatment order – if that was the law's intention. Section 17 was too vague and the judge said it was unlawful.

In Scotland, however, extended leave has not been found unlawful and it is widely used.

Since then critics of community care have argued that many tragic cases of homelessness and deprivation among former psychiatric patients could be prevented by a proper community treatment order. But the idea of nurses barging into people's homes and injecting them forcibly is an unacceptable and unworkable concept. A law that made vulnerable patients attend for supervision and care – but not treatment, unless they consented to it – might be ethical and more widely acceptable.

In 1993, after a widely reported case of an inadequately treated schizophrenic man who climbed into the lions' den at London Zoo and was mauled, the Royal College of Psychiatrists came up with detailed recommendations for a community supervision order. Such an order would last up to six months, could be renewed, and would make patients comply because they could be readmitted compulsorily to hospital if they dropped out of the organized care.

A committee of MPs from all parties, however, said that the government should not take up the Royal College of Psychiatrists' recommendations.[4] Their main argument against the idea was that existing procedures would be more than enough to ensure continuing care if only they were followed properly. These included two further parts of the 1983 Mental Health Act, plus changes to community care that were embodied in the NHS and Community Care Act 1990.

The community care changes are discussed in more detail in the Introduction. Two main points, however, apply to vulnerable patients with long-term mental illness. Firstly, such patients should not be discharged from hospital until a properly coordinated programme of care has been set up. Secondly, the programme should be arranged and coordinated by one key worker or care manager to whom patients, their relatives, and others can turn for help. Thus, these changes allow close supervision of patients at risk. They rely, however, on patients voluntarily accepting help.

The two other parts of the Mental Health Act that already

provide supervision in the community are sections 117 and 7. Section 117 gives patients who are discharged from sections 3, 37, 47, and 48 (see below) the legal right to continuing support from psychiatric and social services until these authorities consider it unnecessary. Section 7 authorizes the appointment of a guardian to supervise care (see below).

If enough money and effort was spent on making sure that all these existing provisions were used properly, nothing extra would be needed, said the MPs' committee. The government, however, set up its own review of mental health law at the same time and recommended two new measures for better supervision of mentally ill people thought to be most at risk: a system of local registration and a new power under the Mental Health Act. Some critics say that putting someone's name on a mental health 'at risk' register infringes civil liberties and others argue that, unless proper community care is available to those on the register, they have little value.

The proposed legal measure – a supervised discharge order – was equally controversial. But it entered the statute books in 1995. It obliges mental health teams to hold urgent review meetings when certain patients (those discharged from hospital under the new order because they are unlikely to keep up with care voluntarily and are very likely to relapse) fail to comply with their agreed programmes of community care. The new order does not include compulsory treatment or readmission to hospital; it merely makes mental health teams think again when things go wrong. Like supervision registers, the supervised discharge order has been criticized for being, on the one hand too Draconian, and on the other, quite toothless.

Section 7: Guardianship   This order offers an alternative to hospital admission in which the patient is looked after by an appointed guardian. This can be someone approved by social services, for example a relative, or the social services department itself. The guardian has the power to make the patient live in a particular place, agree to see doctors and social workers and other staff, and attend for treatment. The order does not, however, make patients have treatment against their will.

Guardianship requires the same eligibility criteria as section 3; it lasts for the same period and offers the same rights of appeal. Orders can be discharged by social services as well as psychiatrists, tribunals, and relatives.

Appointing someone to keep an eye on a vulnerable and ill person and to make sure they take the psychiatric help on offer sounds very sensible. But guardianship is used very rarely, maybe because it could be difficult to enforce and maybe because psychiatrists just don't think to use it. In the year up to March 1992 only 233 guardianship orders were made throughout England and Wales. Yet the government reckons that up to 4000 people a year could benefit from and be eligible for some kind of supervision in the community.

Sections 37, 41 and 47: Hospital orders for offenders Like sections 35 and 36 mentioned above, these relate to patients involved in criminal proceedings. Section 37 is more or less the same as section 3 but is used for people who have been found guilty of imprisonable offences (except murder) and have mental disorders. It can be arranged in court: patients do not have to go to prison first. Section 47 is similar to 37 but it refers to sentenced prisoners who become ill.

The usual time limit of a hospital order can be overruled if the court decides that the patient threatens serious harm to the public. A restriction order under section 41 of the Act is added to the main order. Although this extra restriction can be made for a definite period, it is nearly always made 'without limit of time'. A restricted patient can be discharged only by a Mental Health Tribunal chaired by a senior lawyer or by the Home Office.

Rarely, a person is so mentally disordered at the time of being charged that he is found unfit to plead or is declared not guilty by reason of insanity. In such cases the court can make similar hospital orders under a different Act, the Criminal Procedure Act (1964).

CONSENT TO TREATMENT

Patients' trust that their consent will not be misused or misunderstood is an essential part of their relationships with doctors. Consent to treatment is valid when it is given freely and the patient understands the nature and consequences of what is proposed. The onus is always on the doctor to see that an adequate explanation of the treatment and its consequences is given.

All voluntary patients over the age of 16 have the right to refuse any treatment they do not wish to have, except in emergencies. This means, for example, that a doctor would not be sued for operating on someone who had been seriously injured in an accident, even if the person refused surgery. However, in non-emergency situations, if a doctor touches a patient without permission this may be construed as a form of assault.

The Mental Health Act provides exceptions to this rule, saying that when a person's judgment is altered by mental disorder the law should give permission instead. Formal patients on sections 4,5,7,35,135, and 136 have exactly the same right to refuse treatment as informal patients. Those detained under other sections can be given treatment against their consent in certain circumstances which vary with the type of treatment.

Psychiatric treatments not requiring consent Patients detained under any of the treatment sections of the Act may be given any treatment for mental disorder except electroconvulsive therapy (ECT) and psychosurgery (see below). For practical purposes this leaves only drug treatments, because psychotherapy and behaviour therapy rely on patients' cooperation and cannot be given compulsorily.

Under treatment sections drugs can be given without consent for only three months. After that compulsory treatment can continue only if an independent doctor from the Mental Health Act Commission gives a second opinion agreeing with the prescription. In order to form an opinion the second doctor must interview the patient, a nurse, and another member of staff who is neither a nurse or a doctor but knows the patient. Treatment will be reviewed in this way every three months, even if the patient is on a section for years. Treatment for anything other than mental disorder cannot be given to any patient without his consent, except in a medical emergency.

Section 58: Treatments requiring consent or a second opinion A patient's consent must be given for ECT at any time and for psychiatric drugs beyond three months' prescription. If the patient does not consent, a second opinion must be obtained.

Section 57: Treatments requiring consent and a second opinion
Two types of psychiatric surgical treatment which are used very rarely are dealt with separately by the law because they are particularly controversial. One is psychosurgery, the other is hormone implantation (see p. xxix). The independent doctor must be satisfied that the patient has given fully valid consent and must then form an opinion in the same way as described above.

Section 62: Urgent treatment without consent Psychiatric drugs or ECT can be given in emergencies without consent or second opinions if they are life-saving, or aimed at reducing serious suffering, or preventing serious deterioration or violence.

These regulations about consent may seem confusing. Sarah's story illustrates some of the main points:

> Once she had settled into the ward Sarah felt less worried and managed to eat a bit better. She slept quite well for the first two nights, too. The ward doctor who had interviewed and examined her on the first day had prescribed some tablets, an antidepressant and a mild non-addictive sedative. At first Sarah believed that the treatment was helping her but on the third day she began to worry that it might do her some harm.
>
> Quite quickly, she remembered all her previous worries and felt very unsettled, despite lots of explanation and reassurance from staff. She stopped sleeping, eating, and drinking and was soon looking even worse than when admitted. She refused to take any more drugs.

The doctor was very worried about Sarah's physical state. She looked exhausted and thin and was becoming dehydrated, but she refused to let the doctor check her by taking blood for tests. The consultant psychiatrist decided that Sarah's mental state must be treated urgently to prevent any further deterioration, so he asked her GP and a social worker to see her and consider treatment under section 3.

Section 3 was arranged with the agreement of Sarah's husband. The staff were then authorized to give her treatment even though she did not want it. In vain they tried firm persuasion to get her to take the tablets. Forcible injections were not an option.

After three days the doctors decided that Sarah needed electroconvulsive treatment, so they contacted the Mental Health Act Commission and asked for an independent doctor to give an urgent second opinion. This doctor followed the necessary procedures and agreed with the treatment plan that had been recommended by Sarah's doctors.

Under section 58 Sarah started a course of ECT. After the first treatment she started to eat and drink and was soon out of danger. Six weeks later she was discharged from section 3 and went home, feeling her normal self.

General Rights and Restrictions for Patients in Psychiatric Hospitals

In some ways psychiatry is more respectful of patients' rights than other branches of medicine. Psychiatric staff are often much more aware than their colleagues in general hospitals of the need for confidentiality of information and of the importance of patients' opinions and desires.

In most general hospitals doctors and nurses still do their daily rounds by discussing patients in loud voices at the end of their beds. Involvement of patients in decisions about themselves, even in vital issues like planning whether or not to try resuscitation in the event of sudden death, is rare. Full information about the risks and benefits of certain treatments and tests is not always given to patients before getting their consent. Side rooms where patients can go for private conversations are few and far between.

Psychiatry has had to regulate its ways of practising because the care of people with mental health problems has sometimes been abused in the past. Public expectations of health care and the desire to prosecute doctors and others when things go wrong are both increasing. Perhaps other branches of medicine will eventually need formal frameworks for certain aspects of admission and treatment.

The Mental Health Act provides a framework for compulsory psychiatric admission, treatment, and discharge but does not cover broader aspects of care. But the Mental Health Act Commission produces and regularly updates guidelines – a code of practice – for all aspects of psychiatry. Some of these guidelines suggest minimum acceptable standards for general aspects of hospital care. Some of the most difficult issues that the code covers are summarized in Box 4 and discussed below.

BOX 4

Other civil rights issues in psychiatric hospitals

Security measures

- for violent patients
- for patients who have committed crimes
- for patients who wander

Management of personal affairs

- property and finances
- correspondence
- voting

Access to information

- medical and social work records

> Ability to drive
>
> Restrictions of freedom in the future

Security Measures

FOR VIOLENT PATIENTS

Psychiatric hospitals are not prisons and their staff are not warders. In ordinary local psychiatric hospitals there are now few locked wards – those that remain are for intensive supervision and care of particularly disturbed patients. Despite a patient's initial refusal to be admitted and his belief that he is not ill, he will probably not try to leave hospital or refuse treatment once he has been sectioned. It may be that he feels hopeless or intimidated, but many psychiatric staff say that even the most ill patients with the least insight into their conditions seem to be relieved at being in a safe place.

If a sectioned patient does leave, hospital staff are authorized to try to find him and bring him back, with help from the police if necessary. It may seem stupid to take the drastic step of taking a person into hospital against his will and then fail to keep him. But this shows the difficult dilemma in ensuring that patients get care while trying to preserve the rest of their rights. This open-door policy is not without risks and there have been well-publicized accounts of suicidal or disturbed patients who have left hospital with tragic results, despite being sectioned.

The few locked wards that remain have specific uses. Some offer intensive care for patients who are very disturbed for a few days at the height of a serious mental illness, such as mania. Some are used by patients who have committed crimes while disturbed.

There is a myth, however, that all psychiatric patients are dangerous. Occasionally, disturbed patients do become violent, putting staff, other patients or themselves at risk. In violent incidents staff must consider several points of safety (Box 5). If reassurance and diplomacy fail, practical action may be necessary. In emergencies, staff can use physical restraint and then take the violent person away from the situation to cool off.

BOX 5	**How psychiatric staff are trained to cope with violence**
	• Trying to defuse the situation – 'talking down' the violent person and then dealing with whatever triggered off the incident
	• Respecting the interests and safety of the violent person
	• Protecting others
	• Protecting themselves

On some wards there are special side rooms where a patient can calm down, in seclusion. These are probably the only facilities which fit with the standard idea of asylums, and although these rooms are not padded, they certainly resemble cells. The rooms are barely furnished to avoid self-injury. It is well known that someone can strangle using bed linen or inflict serious injuries by smashing mirrors or glass windows.

In 1993 a report by MIND and Liberty, the National Council for Civil Liberties, said that use of seclusion may go against international conventions on human rights and could even amount to torture. The report also criticized parts of the Mental Health Act and many aspects of care in psychiatric hospitals, saying that standards were often lower than those set for prisons.

Mindful of the potential for abuse of this kind of facility, hospitals require their staff to follow strict guidelines when secluding patients. The start of seclusion must be authorized by a doctor and the patient must be closely observed. The date, time, duration, and circumstances of seclusion must be recorded on special forms which are filed in the patient's notes, with copies sent to the hospital managers.

FOR PATIENTS WHO HAVE COMMITTED CRIMES

If the crime concerned was violent or dangerous to the public, the patient will be admitted to a locked hospital or unit. There are three high-security mental hospitals in England, called special hospitals. They are Broadmoor, Rampton, and Ashworth Hospitals. In each region of England and Wales there are also small units which offer an intermediate level of security.

FOR CONFUSED PATIENTS WHO WANDER

Many elderly people are taken to hospital because they have senile dementia and can no longer be cared for at home. In theory, if such people cannot consent to admission they should be sectioned because this will ensure that their time in hospital will be regularly reviewed. In practice, this is not always done. The dubious justification for not sectioning such patients is either that they will not remember that they are in hospital and will not appeal against being there, or that they are there for their own good.

Once in hospital, a confused elderly person may wander away from the ward or out of the building unless staff can keep a very close eye on him. Locking voluntary patients in for long periods is illegal even if it may be sensible. One way round this is to use two door handles, one placed at the top and the other at the bottom, which must be turned in opposite directions to open the door. This feat combines learning and reasoning abilities with a fair degree of physical agility, faculties that most of the vulnerable patients will have lost. Calling a double-handled door unlocked is really cheating but it is one way of making a ward safe without completely imprisoning its residents.

A less reasonable form of restraint used for patients who tend to wander or fall over is a special type of armchair. This has a tray attached to its front, like that on a child's high chair, providing a surface for eating and other activities. Sadly, the sight of a distressed elderly person trying to push away the imprisoning tray is all too common. It could be avoided if wards were given enough staff to observe and help.

Management of Personal Affairs

PROPERTY AND FINANCES

If a person is in hospital for several weeks the patients' bank will help him look after his finances; for example, sickness benefits can be paid into an account. In addition the National Assistance Act places a general duty upon local social services to protect any movable property of hospital patients. A social worker will go on request to the home of a patient who has been admitted suddenly to hospital and sort out any practical problems like emptying the fridge or putting the dog in kennels.

Some people, whether in hospital or at home, are so mentally or physically unwell that they cannot look after their own affairs. Friends or relatives may help out for short periods on an informal basis, but this often becomes complicated if the person concerned is indefinitely incapable of coping, and, sadly, this kind of arrangement is often abused. Relatives of elderly people with senile dementia sometimes start selling property and spending money, saying that it was to be left to them in the will anyway. It may seem fair to them, but this is wrong. Elderly people's own money is theirs till they die, and their wills are valid only after that. Even if elderly people live in hospital they still need and deserve spending money. And those who need long-term care in nursing homes and old people's homes have to pay for it from their own assets until these fall below a certain threshold value.

Someone who becomes incapable of managing his or her finances and other personal affairs but is still capable of consenting to another person doing so can grant power of attorney to that person. Although this arrangement must be set up by a solicitor while a person's mental capacity is still fairly good, it can carry on after that capacity fails. If the person is already incapable of managing his affairs when the decision is made to appoint someone else to do it, power of attorney cannot be granted. Instead, the court of protection, an office of the Supreme Court, can protect and manage the financial affairs and property of the person. The court appoints a suitable and willing person, often a relative or friend, to act as a receiver. This person has to provide proper accounts to show how the money is being used. The court of protection's costs are deducted from the estate of the person whose affairs are being managed.

CORRESPONDENCE

Most patients in psychiatric hospitals, that is those not on sections, are free to send and receive mail without any interference or censorship. Sectioned patients can receive all their mail but some of their outgoing letters may be intercepted if the people to whom they are addressed do not want them. This protects the addressee, perhaps a celebrity or person in an important public position, if a patient with a mental disorder develops fixed and strange ideas about him and decides to bombard him or her with unwelcome mail. But there is not really any good reason why censorship could not be used at the receiving end.

Patients in special high-security hospitals may have any mail intercepted if it is thought that its receipt is likely to cause distress or danger. This ruling might seem unnecessarily restrictive. One concession is that any patient in any hospital is allowed to write without interference to certain officials (Box 6).

BOX 6

Officials to whom patients in special hospitals may write without interference

- Members of Parliament
- European Commission and Court of Human Rights
- Ombudsmen in Parliament, health services or the local authority
- Lawyers
- Hospital managers (and the health authority)
- Social services and after-care services

- Mental Health Act Commission
- Mental Health Review Tribunals
- Community Health Councils
- Court of Protection

VOTING

If patients are registered on the electoral roll before being sectioned they may still vote. But they cannot enter their names onto the roll while in hospital. This a controversial remnant of a law that barred all patients in mental hospitals from voting.

Voluntary patients can vote. Those who have lived in hospital for years can register to vote by using the address from which they were admitted, or that of a friend or relative, and signing a special form. As long as patients are able to understand this declaration form without explanation, staff are bound to help them register and vote if they want to.

Access to Information

All patients have the right to see any of their own medical records written since November 1991 and any records held on computer before that time. Since 1987 people have been allowed to see their social work records, as long as disclosure is not likely to result in serious harm to others or reveal confidential information about others.

Some patients are distressed by what they find in their notes, usually because their doctors have failed to tell them everything or have misunderstood them. A survey by the Consumers' Association in 1992 of people shown their GP's records found that incurable diseases had not been discussed fully and that untrue assumptions were made, for instance that a patient had suffered incest in the past or that patients were depressed when they weren't. Even people with recognized mental illnesses may not like what they find in their notes: one study showed that only half found reading their notes helpful and more than a quarter found them upsetting.[5]

But other research suggests that initial distress is replaced by long-term improvements in communication between patients and doctors. And the right to see records means that their quality and readability should improve, not least because doctors will plan and maintain records in more patient-friendly formats. Summarized records kept by patients and taken along to every consultation of any kind could be the way forward. These are already used widely for children's notes. Patient-held records have even been shown to work for homeless people with mental illnesses, many of whom do not have GPs but tend to see numerous doctors in different places.[6]

Ability to Drive

There are no direct restrictions on driving for people who have been sectioned but there some which prevent people with serious mental disorders from driving passenger service vehicles like buses and taxis (see Box 7).

BOX 7	**Restrictions on drivers of passenger service vehicles who have been mentally ill**
	People who have taken psychiatric medication must be off it for six months and must be completely well.
	People with mental impairment (handicap) and psychopathic disorder as defined in the Mental Health Act are absolutely excluded from driving these vehicles.
	People with serious mental illnesses like schizophrenia and manic depression and those with alcohol or drug addiction must have been completely well for five years (ten years if the problem has tended to occur regularly).
	These restrictions do not apply to driving private vehicles for personal use.

Restrictions of Freedom in the Future

Sadly, there are many ways in which society tends to discriminate against people who have been sectioned. Mental illness in itself is badly misunderstood and the fact that a person has had to be admitted or treated compulsorily unfortunately implies that he or she must have been particularly ill. One specific effect is restriction of eligibility for visas to certain countries.

Making Complaints about Psychiatric Treatment and Care

Complaining about care in the NHS has become a complicated business over the years, with lots of red tape and several different procedures. For example, a complaint about care by hospital doctors and other staff must be made to the consultant in charge. If the consultant cannot resolve the problem the complaint goes to the senior doctor who coordinates public health policy for the whole region. If that fails, two consultants from somewhere else with no direct involvement in the case must review the problem.

Complaints about general practice go to the family health services authority, the local panel that handles things like medical cards and changing doctors. And complaints that are about hospital services and administrative problems, rather than medical care, are handled by hospitals and health authorities. If they cannot satisfy the patient the complaint can be handed on to the health service ombudsman or watchdog.

All these procedures can lead to inquiries and investigations and to action that puts the problem right locally. Of course, if these procedures are not good enough, if financial compensation is needed, or if criminal acts are involved, complaints can end up in court. But many complainants give up before justice is done because they cannot cope with the baffling and long-winded procedures.

Soon, however, complaining about NHS care and services should be much easier. In 1994 the government proposed a new common system to handle all complaints in just two simple steps: the first by local staff, the second by an independent jury. Both steps should be completed within three months and each has specified time limits.

At the first step the staff directly involved in the complaint or a named complaints officer (usually a hospital manager or a general practice senior partner) would have to respond within 48 hours with an oral apology or explanation. If that was unsatisfactory they would investigate further and explain in writing within three weeks, and, if the complainant was still unhappy with the response, they would hand the problem on to the chief executive of the hospital or general practice service.

Most NHS complaints could be settled at step one. Those that needed further consideration would be referred in step two to an independent panel or jury that included non-medical and non-NHS members. The panel would have five weeks to deal with each complaint. At the end of that any doctor or other member of staff judged to have breached professional codes would be referred to the relevant regulatory body, such as the General Medical Council. And, finally, the very few complaints that were still unresolved would be sent on to the health ombudsman, an independent assessor who reports to parliament about failings in the NHS.

Getting Further Information and Advice

The mental health charity MIND has a team of legal experts to campaign for and advise people who may encounter the Mental Health Act. They have published an excellent series of leaflets on the law, the MIND Rights Guides, which are available from MIND's head office in London. That address, and those of other organizations concerned with legal aspects of mental health, are given in Appendix 2.

Glossary – Explaining The Jargon

Abnormal illness behaviour
when psychological problems
are masked by physical
symptoms that have no
apparent physical cause, e.g. in
hysteria and Munchausen's
syndrome.

Acetylcholine a chemical
messenger in the brain and
nervous system that tells nerve
cells what to do.

Acute confusional state a
sudden and brief episode of
disorientation, muddled
thinking, and disturbed
behaviour.

Acute illness an illness of rapid
onset and, usually, of short
duration. The term acute does
not relate to severity of illness.
See *chronic illness*.

Addiction see *drug dependence*.

Affect This is another word for
mood.

Affective disorders disorders of
mood: depression,
hypomania, and mania.

Agoraphobia a fear of being in
public places that causes
anxiety and a desire to avoid
such places. See *phobia*.

Acquired immunodeficiency

syndrome (AIDS) a disease in
which the body's defences
against infection and cancer
are lost. It is caused by the
human immunodeficiency
virus (HIV).

**Alcohol dependence or addiction
(alcoholism)** when alcohol
induces repeated use, partly
because an unpleasant
withdrawal syndrome occurs
when alcohol use is stopped.

Alzheimer's disease a form of
dementia with a slow, steady
onset and with characteristic
abnormalities in the brain.

Amnesia memory loss.

Angiography injecting dye into
blood vessels and taking X-
rays to see the state of the
vessels that the dye shows up.
Angiography can be used to
investigate whether the blood
supply to the brain is
disrupted.

Anorectic (anorexic) a label
used to describe someone with
anorexia nervosa.

Anorexia a general medical
term meaning loss of appetite.

Anorexia nervosa a disorder
characterized by persistent and

usually secretive self-
starvation, with loss of at least
one-quarter of normal body
weight, hormonal imbalances
including period problems, and
other physical effects of
starvation.

Anticholinergic drugs drugs
that counteract the side effects
(shaking, stiffness) of
antipsychotic drugs.

Antidepressant drugs drugs
that alleviate depression.

Antipsychotic drugs also called
neuroleptics and major
tranquillizers, these drugs
relieve hallucinations,
delusions, and severe agitation
in psychotic illnesses such as
schizophrenia.

Anxiety the group of feelings
and experiences that occur at
times of acute stress:
nervousness, fear, worrying,
irritability, sweating,
breathlessness, 'butterflies',
and racing pulse.

Anxiety management training
group therapy for treating
anxiety in which the therapist
explains the symptoms of
anxiety and shows how to deal
with and prevent them.

Anxiety state a disorder in
which anxiety symptoms are
sufficiently severe to make the
sufferer feel ill, often with
tiredness and insomnia too.

Anxiolytic drug a drug that
dispels or lessens anxiety.

Approved social worker (ASW)
a social worker with special
training in the use of the

Mental Health Act, the law that
authorizes compulsory
psychiatric care and treatment.

Asylum literally, a place of
safety. In the past its use to
describe psychiatric institutions
has led to stigma, and the term
now has an unwarranted
meaning of 'madhouse'.

Auditory hallucination an
hallucination of a sound,
usually a voice. See
hallucination.

Baby blues transient episode of
tearfulness and irritability in the
first week after childbirth.

Behaviour therapy an 'action
cure' in which a therapist,
usually a clinical psychologist,
helps a patient to examine
problematic behaviour patterns
and change them for the better.

Benzodiazepines a group of
sedative and tranquillizing
drugs such as diazepam
(Valium), now prescribed to
treat insomnia and anxiety only
for short periods because long-
term use can lead to addiction.

Bereavement the psychological
response to a severe loss,
usually the death of a loved
one.

Beta-blocking drugs drugs
used to treat anxiety and
panic. They stop the body's
chemical messengers from
transmitting symptoms of
anxiety and panic, and thereby
reduce their effects.

Bipolar affective disorder see
manic depression.

Blunting (flattening) of

emotions an emotional disorder in which the ability to express and respond to emotions becomes limited. It occurs most commonly in schizophrenia.

Borderline personality disorder a personality disorder in which very transient but disturbing symptoms of mental illness occur. See *personality disorder*.

Brief recurrent depression a problem with frequent episodes of serious and disabling depression that last only a few days.

Bulimia nervosa a psychological disorder in which the sufferer secretly has huge eating binges and then induces vomiting or uses laxatives to avoid weight gain.

Cardiomyopathy a disorder in which the heart muscle degenerates, causing decreased stamina, breathlessness, and sometimes premature death. One of several causes of cardiomyopathy is prolonged heavy alcohol use.

Care manager a coordinator employed by social services to arrange and buy packages of social help and community care for needy clients or patients.

Catatonia a severe, acute, state characterized by reduced alertness and either statue-like immobility or marked agitation. It was once a common feature of schizophrenia but is rare now, presumably because modern treatments prevent it.

Chromosomes paired packages of genes present in all the body's cells. Humans usually have 23 pairs including a pair of sex chromosomes: XX in women and XY in men. See *gene*.

Chronic fatigue syndrome (also known as myalgic encephalomyelitis, ME) a long-term problem of lethargy, tiredness, and muscle aching on exertion.

Chronic illness illness of long duration. The term does not relate to severity. See *acute illness*.

Cirrhosis a severe and irreversible inflammation and scarring disease of the liver, caused particularly (though not exclusively) by prolonged and heavy alcohol use.

Cognitive impairment impairment of orientation (for time, place, or person), awareness, intellect or memory.

Cognitive behaviour therapy (cognitive therapy) a kind of mental retraining in positive thinking, in which the therapist shows the patient that ways of thinking when ill may lead to a misleading view of the world and may negatively influence emotions and psychological symptoms.

Cognitive theory the notion that certain patterns of thinking precede, cause, and perpetuate certain mental health problems including depression and the eating disorders anorexia and bulimia nervosa.

Community care continuing care outside hospital (including psychiatric and medical care and social help) for people who would otherwise need to live in hospital.

Community meeting a group meeting, perhaps of all patients on a ward or all residents in a hostel, to discuss issues that affect everyone present.

Community mental health centre a facility like a general practice health centre catering solely for people with mental health problems.

Community psychiatric nurse (CPN) a nurse who works outside hospital, visiting patients in their own homes and hostels.

Compulsion an unwelcome and unwarranted urge to perform a certain action.

Compulsive eating a disorder in which the sufferer feels that eating is out of personal control. The main features are being preoccupied by food and dieting, eating when not hungry, and hating oneself. It is often associated with obesity.

Compulsory admission or treatment admission or treatment, under the Mental Health Act, of a disturbed patient who refuses to accept psychiatric help.

Computed tomography (CT or CAT scanning) using X-rays guided by a computer to give pictures in sequential 'slices'. CT can be used to illustrate the structure of the brain.

Conduct disorder a pattern of persistently antisocial behaviour in a child, more than simple naughtiness or disobedience.

Counselling one kind of 'talking cure' in which clients are given the chance to explore their feelings and find personal and practical solutions to their problems.

Court of Protection an office of the Supreme Court that can protect and manage the financial affairs and property of a person who is so incapacitated that he or she is unable to understand the meaning of or make a decision on granting power of attorney.

Creutzfeld-Jakob disease a rare, rapidly progressive presenile dementia caused by infection with a small virus-like particle called a prion.

Crisis intervention urgent mental health assessment and help, usually by a team of health and social work professionals who visit the home of someone with a mental health crisis to try to avert a full scale emergency.

CT scanning see *computed tomography*.

Deliberate self-harm A non-fatal act such as a drug overdose or wrist-cutting. It means the same as parasuicide.

Delirium an acute and fluctuating state of confusion with disorientation and drowsiness, usually caused by a transient event in the brain such as infection, drug toxicity, or a small stroke.

Delirium tremens (DT's) severe confusion, often with psychotic symptoms and fits, in an alcohol-dependent person who is abruptly withdrawing from alcohol in the absence of a safe substitute and medical supervision.

Delusion a belief or idea that is demonstrably false, is not explained by the person's past experiences, and cannot be shaken by logical argument. Delusions occur in psychotic illnesses like schizophrenia and manic depression.

Dementia a progressive state of confusion, with intellectual and other types of mental deterioration that end in death. See *Alzheimer's disease, multi-infarct dementia,* and *presenile dementia.*

Depot injections long-acting forms of antipsychotic drugs, injected every few weeks into a muscle, usually the buttock, which provide a constant steady dose and reduce the need to take daily tablets.

Depression sustained episode of low mood that interferes with normal emotional, and sometimes social and physical, functioning.

Desensitization a kind of exposure therapy in which an anxious, phobic, or obsessional patient is gradually exposed to the anxiety-provoking stimulus and taught how to cope with the anxiety by relaxation.

Drug any chemical, whether natural or man-made, taken for some specific effect.

Drug dependence or addiction when a drug induces repeated use, partly because an unpleasant withdrawal syndrome occurs when drug use is stopped.

Drug holiday stopping long-term medication temporarily under close medical supervision, to give the body a break.

Drying out (detoxification) stopping alcohol or drug abuse abruptly under medical supervision, while taking gradually reducing doses of a safer substitute to lessen or abolish withdrawal symptoms.

Eating disorders abnormal patterns of eating that cause physical problems and include anorexia nervosa, bulimia nervosa, and compulsive eating.

Electroconvulsive therapy (ECT) a treatment in which a small electric current is passed through the brain of an anaesthetized and relaxed patient (usually someone with severe depression) to induce a fit and alleviate psychiatric symptoms.

Electroencephalography (EEG)

a tracing of the brain's electrical signals.

Empowerment giving individuals and groups facts and advice so that they can express their wishes and needs more effectively and make more informed choices.

Endogenous depression depression that occurs spontaneously and is caused by an inherent tendency, e.g. a chemical imbalance in the brain.

Enzymes a family of chemicals that act as catalysts for nearly all of the body's chemical reactions. In alcohol abuse the enzymes in the liver are overproduced and can be detected in the blood at unusually high concentrations.

Exposure therapy a kind of behaviour therapy in which an anxious, obsessional, or phobic patient is helped to face a distressing stimulus. Examples are desensitization and flooding.

Expressed emotion the level of emotion within a group of people, usually a family. Research has shown that families with high levels of expressed emotion tend to lead to early relapse in schizophrenic patients living at home.

Family therapy psychotherapy in which the whole family attends together to look at abnormal patterns of communication and behaviour that have made at least one member of the family psychiatrically ill or disturbed.

Fight or flight response how the body responds to acute stress. See *anxiety*.

First rank symptoms certain symptoms that are strongly suggestive of schizophrenia and help in diagnosing it, such as the unwarranted feeling that thoughts and behaviour are completely controlled by an external force.

Fitness to plead a legal term describing the defendant's mental ability to understand court proceedings and to plead guilty or not guilty.

Flight of ideas an abnormally quick rate of thinking that is difficult to follow, occurring in mania and hypomania.

Flooding therapy a kind of exposure therapy in which an anxious, obsessional or phobic patient has to face a distressing stimulus in its full extent, with support from a therapist.

Forensic psychiatry the psychiatric speciality concerned with criminal behaviour and mental health law.

Gene a coded chemical sequence on a chromosome that acts as a blueprint for the body's building blocks – and thereby for the body's appearance and function – and passes on heritable characteristics to the next generation. See *chromosome*.

Group home lightly supervised

accommodation shared by several people with similar mental health problems and similar needs for minimal social care.

Guardianship a power under the Mental Health Act that allows an appointed guardian to look after a patient who would otherwise need compulsory admission to hospital.

Hallucination an experience of one of the five senses (hearing, vision, taste, smell, touch) which is perceived as real but has no external cause.

Hallucinogenic drug a drug that causes hallucinations.

History your personal story that explains how and, to a certain extent, why you need help. Doctors, nurses, social workers and other staff may all need to 'take' your history by interviewing you. They will ask questions about your life, relationships, work, and any past or present problems.

Histrionic behaviour overdramatic behaviour.

Hormones chemical messengers that are made in glands and that tell parts of the body what to do.

Human immunodeficiency virus (HIV) the virus that causes AIDS, the acquired immune deficiency syndrome.

Huntington's disease (Huntington's chorea) an exclusively hereditary form of pre-senile dementia with a characteristic disorder of movement.

Hypertension high blood pressure.

Hyperventilation excessively quick breathing when anxious that can cause a chemical imbalance in the body, with further frightening symptoms.

Hypnotic drug another name for a sedative.

Hypochondria a persistent tendency to be overly concerned about health and illness.

Hypomania a common and slightly reduced form of mania. True mania is very severe and the term is rarely used. This terminology probably reflects the fact that modern treatments have lessened the severity of most episodes.

Hysteria a rare disruption of bodily function that initially seems due to physical illness but has no identifiable physical cause and is really caused by powerful psychological stress that cannot be expressed any other way.

Informal patient see *voluntary patient*.

Insight degree of understanding. In psychiatry this usually refers to a patient's ability to recognize that he or she is ill.

Insomnia inability to sleep.

Korsakoff's psychosis permanent brain damage with marked memory loss caused by lack of the B vitamin thiamine, usually resulting from heavy alcohol use. It is closely related to and usually preceded by *Wernicke's encephalopathy* (see below).

Learning disabilities intellectual impairment starting early in life, usually before or around the time of birth. People with learning disabilities were previously called mentally handicapped.

Lithium a naturally occurring element. In the form of lithium salts it stabilizes mood swings and alleviates mania and severe depression.

Major tranquillizers see antipsychotic drugs.

Mania very severe and persistent elevation of mood – beyond normal happiness – accompanied by restlessness, irritability, and psychosis. See *hypomania*, which is the commoner term.

Manic depression (manic depressive psychosis) a serious mental illness with severe swings of mood which can last many months. Episodes of illness are usually of depression or mania (often hypomania) but not both at the same time. Manic depression is also called bipolar affective disorder.

Mental handicap see *learning disabilities*.

Mental Health Act the law that, within strict criteria, allows removal to a place of safety, assessment, and treatment of any disturbed adult who refuses psychiatric help but seems to need it.

Mental Health Act Commission the legal body that supervises the use of the Mental Health Act and considers and makes recommendations on wide aspects of mental welfare.

Mental Health Review Tribunal an independent body that hears cases for and against the use of the Mental Health Act.

Mental state examination an examination of your state of mind, made by observing your behaviour and mood and by listening carefully to your answers to specific questions about psychiatric symptoms.

Misidentification syndrome this occurs mainly in dementia, when the sufferer muddles up reality with memories and misinterpretations of events.

Mood-stabilizing drugs drugs used in manic depression, for example lithium and carbamazepine.

Monoamine oxidase inhibitors (MAOIs) a family of antidepressant drugs, rarely prescribed now because serious side effects can occur if certain foods or other drugs are taken. Their name reflects their action on certain brain chemicals.

Multi-infarct dementia a senile dementia caused by successive small strokes.

Multiple personality a very rare

personality disorder in which the sufferer invents several completely different personalities.

Munchausen's syndrome a personality disorder in which the sufferer fakes real illness, apparently to gain attention and transient admission to hospital.

Munchausen's syndrome by proxy when a person with a personality disorder causes fake signs of illness in someone else, usually in a child.

Myalgic encephalomyelitis (ME) see *chronic fatigue syndrome*.

Nearest relative the relative who, as defined under the Mental Health Act, has special powers and rights concerning the patient's care.

Negative symptoms those aspects of chronic schizophrenia that make sufferers withdrawn and reduce their emotional depth and warmth. See *positive symptoms*.

Nervous breakdown disruptive mental health problems that interfere with sufferers' lives. Doctors and other mental health professionals do not usually use this term because it is so vague and does not detail the kind of problems suffered.

Neuroleptic see *antipsychotic drugs*.

Neurosis a psychiatric disorder in which the symptoms are like exaggerations of normal experience and the patient

does not lose touch with reality. The term is outdated now because it is too vague and is often used derogatively in non-medical language.

Neurotic depression depression without psychotic symptoms.

Neurotransmitters chemical messengers in the brain and nervous system that tell nerve cells what to do.

Nihilistic delusions extremely negative delusions in severe psychotic depression: sufferers believe that things, e.g. parts of their own body, no longer work or even exist.

Nuclear magnetic resonance imaging (NMR) using strong magnetic fields to make parts of the body's atoms spin, giving off radio waves that can be built into a picture of the organ scanned, for example the brain.

Obesity when a person is overweight for their height or is more than one-fifth above the normal weight range for height. See *compulsive eating*.

Obsession a spontaneous intrusive thought that causes anxiety.

Obsessive-compulsive disorder a disorder related to anxiety in which unwelcome worries intrude into ordinary thinking and compel the sufferer to take particular actions.

Occupational therapist a non-medical specialist trained and qualified at college or university to help patients back to self-confidence and independence and to restore their skills, including everyday ones like shopping and cooking, that may be lost during illness.

Opiate drugs drugs derived from opium poppies including heroin, morphine, and codeine.

Organic mental illness a disorder caused by demonstrably impaired functioning of the brain.

Pancreatitis inflammation of the pancreas (a digestive organ) caused particularly, though not exclusively, by heavy alcohol use.

Panic attack when anxiety occurs suddenly and severely.

Panic disorder a kind of anxiety state in which the sufferer has repeated and disabling panic attacks.

Paranoia this term has had a wide range of meanings in the history of psychiatry but is now used to describe strong feelings or delusions of persecution.

Parasuicide an apparent attempt to commit suicide that may, rather, be a call for attention and help. See *deliberate self-harm*.

Passivity a delusion that one's own actions are directly controlled by some outside person or force, as if one is a puppet.

Peripheral neuropathy numbness, tingling, or burning in the feet caused by lack of B vitamins such as

thiamine. It commonly occurs among heavy drinkers because alcohol blocks absorption of these vitamins.

Personality the combination of characteristic features – including temperament, emotional responses, intellect, sociability, attitudes – that makes individuals.

Personality disorder an abnormality of personal functioning giving rise to ingrained behaviour, attitudes, and emotional responses that cause suffering to the self or others and impair social function.

Phenothiazines one family of antipsychotic drugs.

Phobia an unbearable fear of a particular situation that would not normally bother most people. The resulting anxiety is so severe that it can be dealt with only by avoiding the frightening situation.

Pick's disease a presenile dementia that particularly affects the frontal lobes of the brain and affects personality first.

Positive symptoms those aspects of chronic schizophrenia that are florid and active, e.g. hallucinations, delusions, thought disorder. See *negative symptoms*.

Positron emission tomography (PET scanning) giving a minute dose of a radioactive substance that combines with brain chemicals and allows detection by a scanner, showing up the distribution of brain chemicals.

Postnatal (or postpartum) psychiatric illness psychiatric illness – usually depression, occasionally psychosis – that follows childbirth.

Post-traumatic stress disorder a kind of mixed anxious, phobic, and depressive state that follows a sudden, severe stress such as assault, battle, or mass disaster. The symptoms include vivid and persistent re-experiencing of the traumatic event, through intrusive memories, images, and dreams.

Power of attorney the power invested in a nominated person to manage the financial affairs and property of a person who is incapacitated because of illness (usually mental illness) but is able to understand the meaning of and need for the transfer of power.

Premenstrual syndrome irritability, moodiness, bloating, and breast tenderness for up to two weeks before each period.

Presenile dementias a group of dementias that tend to occur before old age. They include *Pick's disease, Creutzfeld-Jakob disease* and *Huntington's disease*.

Primary care care from a GP and his or her team.

Prophylaxis measures taken to prevent illness.

Pseudo-Cushing's syndrome a disorder of the adrenal glands causing obesity and puffiness, sex hormone imbalances, and excess hairiness. It can occur in alcohol abusers.

Pseudodementia a reversible state in elderly patients that appears to be a chronic confusional state, mimicking dementia, but is really a severe form of depression.

Psychiatrist a medical doctor who has trained and specialized in psychiatry.

Psychiatry the branch of medicine concerned with mental health diagnosis, treatment, and care.

Psychoanalysis a kind of psychotherapy in which the therapist interprets the client's or patient's problems with reference to a certain school of mental philosophy, such as that of Freud or Jung.

Psychogeriatric services services specially for elderly people with mental health problems.

Psychological or psychometric tests quizzes and exercises that test memory, intelligence, personality, perception, capability for abstract thinking and other mental functions.

Psychologist a non-medical specialist with a degree in psychology. Clinical psychologists, who work with psychiatric teams, have had specialized postgraduate training in the thought and behaviour patterns of people with mental health problems.

Psychology the social science that studies and can alter human behaviour.

Psychomotor retardation marked slowing of the mind and body that can occur in severe depression.

Psychopathy (psychopathic personality disorder) a severe and persistent tendency to behave antisocially and irresponsibly. See *personality disorder* and *conduct disorder*.

Psychosexual problems mixed emotional and physical problems that impair sexual performance.

Psychosis a mental disorder in which there is a break from everyday reality with symptoms that differ widely from most people's experience, such as hallucinations and delusions.

Psychosurgery operating on the brain to alleviate severe psychiatric illness or very troublesome personality traits. Rarely performed now and, when it is done, it usually involves small cuts in the brain made under X-ray guidance.

Psychotherapy a 'talking cure' in which problems can be alleviated by a therapist who provides a trustworthy, trusting, and confiding relationship and explores past experiences.

Psychotic relating to or suffering from psychosis.

Psychotic depression a severe form of depression with psychotic features such as hallucinations and delusions.

Psychotropic drug any drug taken to affect mental function.

Reactive depression depression that develops in response to a defined stress.

Relaxation training in which the signs of muscular tension are highlighted and a system of progressively relaxing exercises are taught.

Remission the healthy or relatively healthy gap between attacks of a relapsing illness.

Respite care short-stay residential care for patients with disability and high dependency on others, so that the patient's usual carers at home can have some time off.

Response prevention a behaviour therapy technique for compulsive patients. The therapist helps the patient to overcome the urge to perform a compulsive act, initially by delaying the action, eventually by stopping it altogether.

Responsible medical officer (RMO) the doctor, usually consultant, in charge of the care of a patient being detained or treated under the Mental Health Act.

Ritual (compulsive ritual) an entrenched pattern of senseless compulsive acts. See *obsessive-compulsive disorder*.

Schizoid personality an odd, introspective, emotionally detached personality type.

Schizophrenia a serious mental illness characterized by psychosis – hallucinations, delusions, disturbed thinking – and by problems with behaviour and emotional responses.

Seasonal affective disorder a form of depression that regularly occurs in winter and improves in spring.

Section part of the Mental Health Act. Rather than saying 'detain or treat under a section of the act', psychiatric staff often use the lazy slang verb 'to section'. It has replaced the verb 'to certify'.

Selective serotonin reuptake inhibitors (SSRIs) a family of antidepressant drugs which act on the neurotransmitter serotonin in the brain and thereby elevate mood.

Senile dementia dementia starting in old age.

Sensate focus therapy a behaviour therapy for psychosexual problems, involving a series of graded tasks or exercises.

Serotonin a chemical messenger in the brain that is thought to be deficient in people with depression.

Signs objective features of illness that may be externally obvious or may be detected by medical examinations and tests. A rash is an example of a medical sign. See *symptoms*.

Single photon emission computed tomography
(SPECT) a recent variant of CT scanning that may be used to investigate brain disease.

Social phobia a fear of meeting people in social situations, which leads to anxiety and a desire to avoid others. See *phobia*.

Social skills training group therapy in which the therapist explains body language and other social communication and shows how to feel more confident.

Social worker non-medical professionals trained and qualified at university or college to understand all aspects of social welfare. Psychiatric social workers have had special postgraduate training in mental health problems and approved social workers are qualified to use mental health laws.

Somatization a failure to recognize and deal with emotional stress and to express it instead as generalized physical symptoms.

Special hospital a high-security hospital for mentally ill or disturbed criminal offenders.

Stroke Death of part of the brain, caused by lack of blood supply because a blood vessel in the brain has ruptured or been blocked by a spasm or clot. Small strokes can cause *multi-infarct dementia*.

Symptoms features of illness that are experienced by sufferers but may not necessarily be obvious externally or detectable by medical examination and tests. Headache is an example.

Syndrome a collection of symptoms and signs which together make a distinct and recognizable health problem, a syndrome. See *symptoms* and *signs*.

Suicide self-killing. See also *parasuicide* and *deliberate self-harm*.

Tardive dyskinesia a brain disorder that causes abnormal involuntary body movements such as repetitive and unnecessary chewing. It tends to occur in people who have taken antipsychotic drugs for prolonged periods.

Therapeutic community places where people with similar mental health problems meet together for group therapy every day and may live together if the unit is residential. The community is run democratically and members are expected to assume communal responsibilities.

Thiamine a vitamin in the B group that is important for a healthy brain and nervous system and whose absorption is blocked by alcohol. It is commonly lacking in people who abuse alcohol. See *Wernicke's encephalopathy* and *Korsakoff's psychosis*.

Thought disorder the irrational, muddled and characteristically strange thinking that occurs in psychotic illnesses,

particularly in schizophrenia and mania.

Transference the process by which a patient or client in psychotherapy develops feelings for and attitudes to the therapist that were initially experienced in a previous important relationship, for example with a parent.

Tricyclic drugs a family of antidepressant drugs. Their name reflects the shape of the molecules that make up their chemical structure.

Unconscious mind that part of the mind that, according to Freud, we are unaware of but are controlled by for much of the time. Psychoanalysis is usually directed at the unconscious mind.

Unipolar affective disorder a mental illness with severe episodes of either mania or depression, in which the mood always swings in the same direction.

Unit of alcohol a measure of alcohol consumption that allows comparison of different types of alcohol use. One unit is equal to one standard measure of spirits, vermouth, or fortified wine; one glass of wine; or half a pint of beer.

Volatile substance abuse (glue sniffing) inhalation of volatile substances such as certain glues, lighter fuel, and nail polish to achieve similar effects to those of alcohol.

Voluntary (or informal) patient

a patient who has chosen to accept psychiatric assessment, care or treatment and has not been subjected to legal compulsion under the Mental Health Act.

Ward doctor the doctor who works most regularly on any given ward, usually a senior house officer or registrar – both of whom are doctors in postgraduate training.

Ward round a meeting held by doctors, nurses, and other mental health staff to discuss the progress of patients on the ward. Patients are often invited into the meeting, one at a time, to join the discussion.

Wernicke's encephalopathy a sudden severe brain disease caused by deficiency of the B vitamin thiamine, most commonly because of prolonged alcohol use. The symptoms include severe confusion, loss of balance and double vision, even when sober. See *Korsakoff's psychosis*.

Help Yourself – Advisory and Self-Help Organizations

Most of these organizations have already been mentioned in this book. Here are the detailed addresses:

GENERAL ADVICE

MIND (National Association for Mental Health)
Granta House
15–19 Broadway
London E15 4BQ
Tel.: 0181 519 2122

MIND has a long history of successful campaigning (for example, for a better mental health law) and providing support and advice for people in mental distress. Around 200 local groups nationwide are affiliated to MIND and provide friendship, advice, advocacy, day care and accommodation. MIND has an extensive list of publications on all aspects of mental health.

SANELINE
Tel.: 0171 724 8000 (2 p.m. till midnight, daily)

For anyone facing a mental health crisis, a helpline offering support and information including details of local mental health organizations. SANE has an extensive and up to date computerized database of mental health services throughout Britain, both statutory (NHS and social services) and voluntary.

Mental Health Foundation
37 Mortimer Street
London W1N 7RJ
Tel.: 0171 580 0145

The only fundraising, grant-giving and campaigning charity for both mental illness and learning disability in the UK.

The Richmond Fellowship
8 Addison Road
London W14 6DL
Tel.: 0171 603 6373

The fellowship runs a nationwide network of homes and therapeutic communities for people whose mental health problems make living independently difficult.

Mental After Care Association
25 Bedford Square
London WC1B 3HW
Tel.: 0171 436 6194

The association offers a wide

range of services in the community, including accommodation, for people with mental health problems. It also provides information and support for carers.

Carers National Association
20–25 Glasshouse Yard
London EC1A 4JS
Tel.: 0171 490 8818

All too often, family members and friends who provide care for mentally ill and disabled people do not themselves get any support. This association campaigns for, advises, and supports carers nationwide.

MENCAP (The Royal Society for Mentally Handicapped Children and Adults) national centre
123 Golden Lane
London EC1 0RT
Tel.: 0171 454 0454

MENCAP offers support, information, and education to people with learning disabilities and their carers. It also campaigns nationally for better research and services.

COUNSELLING AND PSYCHOTHERAPY

These associations have registers of counsellors and psychotherapists nationwide:

British Association of Counselling
1 Regent Place
Rugby
Warwickshire CV21 2PJ

Tel.: 01788 578328

National Council of Psychotherapists and Hypnotherapy Register
46 Oxhey Road
Watford
Hertfordshire WD1 4QQ
Tel.: 01923 227772

ANXIETY AND INSOMNIA

Relaxation for Living
168–170 Oatlands Drive
Weybridge
Surrey KT13 9ET
Tel.: 01932 831000

Advice and information on relaxation training, including a range of audiotapes.

Insomnia Self-Help Group
10 Barley Mow Passage
London W4 4PH
Tel.: 0181 994 9874 (5–10 p.m. Monday to Friday)

This group offers support and a quarterly newsletter.

PHOBIAS

Two self-help groups that offer support:

Phobic Action
Hornbeam House, Claybury Grounds
Manor Road
Woodford Green
Essex IG8 8PR
Tel.: 0181 559 2459

Phobics Society
4 Cheltenham Road
Chorlton-Cum-Hardy
Manchester M21 1QN
Tel.: 0161 881 1937

The Maudsley Hospital
Denmark Hill
London SE5 8AZ
Tel.: 0171 703 6333

The Maudsley Hospital provides information on and treatment of phobias.

RELATIONSHIP PROBLEMS

Relate
National Office
Herbert Gray College
Little Church Street
Rugby
Warwickshire CV21 3AP
Tel.: 01788 573241

Relate offers counselling on a wide range of relationship problems. Its many local branches are listed in phone books and local services directories.

Gay and Lesbian Switchboard
London area
Tel.: 0171 837 7324 (24 hours)

Most large towns and cities have local support helplines for gay people, listed in phone and local directories.

PYCHOSEXUAL PROBLEMS

Family Planning Information Service
27–35 Mortimer Street
London W1N 7RJ
Tel.: 0171 636 7866

As well as family planning, the service offers psychosexual counselling and treatment.

DEPRESSION AND MANIC DEPRESSION

Fellowship of Depressives Anonymous
36 Chestnut Avenue
Beverley
North Humberside HU17 9QU
Tel.: 01482 860619

A self-help organization that puts sufferers in touch with each other, via groups and a penfriend scheme.

Depressives Associated
PO Box 1022
London SE1 7BQ
Tel.: 0181 760 0544 (answering machine)

This organization provides information and support for users and carers through self-help groups.

Manic Depression Fellowship
8–10 High Street
Kingston-Upon-Thames
Surrey KT1 1EY
Tel.: 0181 974 6550

The fellowship, which has local branches, supports and advises both sufferers and their families. It also supports research and aims to educate the public and caring professions.

POSTNATAL PROBLEMS

National Childbirth Trust
Alexandra House, Oldham Terrace
Acton
London W3 6NH
Tel.: 0181 992 8637

The trust offers support, friendship, and education to parents before and after the birth of a child and will try to help with any problems of early parenthood.

Association of Post-Natal Illness
25 Jerdan Place
London SW6 1BE
Tel.: 0171 386 0868

The association can put depressed mothers in touch with others who have had similar experiences. It also provides information on postnatal problems.

National Council for One-Parent Families
255 Kentish Town Road
London NW5 2LX
Tel.: 0171 267 1361

The council can help with practical, financial, and legal problems of single parenthood. *See **Bereavement** section (below) for organizations that support and inform bereaved parents.*

BEREAVEMENT

CRUSE Bereavement Care
Cruse House
126 Sheen Road
Richmond
Surrey TW9 1UR
Tel.: 0181 940 4818

Offers advice and information and, through local branches, support for bereaved people.

Lesbian and Gay Bereavement Project
Unitarian Rooms,
Hoop Lane
London NW11 0RL
Tel.: 0181 455 8894

Terrence Higgins Trust
52–54 Grays Inn Road
London WC1X 8JU
Tel.: 0171 831 0330

Both the above offer support, counselling, and information about bereavement and AIDS.

Compassionate Friends
53 North Street
Bristol BS3 1EN
Tel.: 01179 292778

An international organization of bereaved parents that offers friendship, support, information and counselling to parents who have lost a child of any age. It has two specialized branches – Parents of Murdered Children and Shadow of Suicide (for parents whose children have died by suicide).

The following organizations offer support and information to parents whose babies have died, as well as prompting and funding research:

Foundation for the Study of Infant Deaths
35 Belgrave Square
London SW1X 8QB
Tel.: 0171 235 1721 (cot death helpline)

The Stillbirth and Neonatal Death Society (SANDS)
28 Portland Place
London W1N 4DE
Tel.: 0171 436 5881

Cot Death Society
116 Alt Road
Formby
Merseyside L37 8BW
Tel.: 01704 870005

Miscarriage Association
Clayton Hospital
Northgate
Wakefield WF1 3JS
Tel.: 01924 200799 (24-hour answering machine)

SCHIZOPHRENIA

National Schizophrenia Fellowship
28 Castle Street
Kingston Upon Thames
Surrey KT1 15S
Tel.: 0181 547 3937
Advice line: 0181 974 6814

The fellowship is the largest support group in Britain for people with schizophrenia and their families, with several regional headquarters and more than 100 local groups. As well as support, the fellowship offers information and advice (including leaflets, reports, and a newsletter) on treatment, services, and research. It campaigns for better services and raises money for research.

SANE (Schizophrenia – A National Emergency)
199–205 Old Marylebone Road
London NW1 5QP
Tel.: 0171 724 6520

SANELINE
(Crisis phoneline
2 p.m.–midnight daily)
Tel.: 0171 724 8000

SANE is a campaigning organization that raises funds for research into schizophrenia and for services for sufferers and their families. It also aims to raise awareness of the problems of schizophrenia and other mental illnesses and the need for better services.

Schizophrenia Association of Great Britain
International Schizophrenia Centre
Bryn Hyfryd, The Crescent
Bangor, Gwynnedd
Wales LL57 2AG
Tel.: 01248 354048 or 670379

DEMENTIA AND OLD-AGE PROBLEMS

Alzheimer's Disease Society
10 Greencoat Place
London SW1P 1PH
Tel.: 0181 306 0606

The society provides support and information, including a range of explanatory leaflets. It also supports research.

Huntington's Disease Association
108 Battersea High Street
London SW11 3HP
Tel.: 0171 223 7000

The association offers a wide range of services to around 6000 members. These services include local support groups, advice and education, counselling about predictive testing, a research programme, a welfare fund, and a respite care home.

Age Concern Greater London
Astral House
1268 London Road
London SW16 4ER
Tel.: 0181 679 8000

Help the Aged
St James Walk
Clerkenwell
London EC1R 0BE
Tel.: 0171 253 0253
  : 01446 745049 (Wales)
  : 0131 556 4666 (Scotland)
  : 01232 230666 (Northern Ireland)

Age Concern and Help the Aged campaign for and support elderly people and their carers – this includes provision of many local services.

The Relatives' Association
5 Tavistock Place
London WC1H 9SS
Tel.: 0171 916 6055

Support and information for relatives and carers of elderly people living in old peoples' and nursing homes.

ALCOHOL AND DRUG PROBLEMS

Alcoholics Anonymous
(London regional and general service office)
11 Redcliffe Gardens
London SW10 9BG
Tel.: 0171 352 3001
or:

AA Great Britain
PO Box 1
Stonebow House
Stonebow
York YO1 2NJ
Tel.: 01904 644026

A national network of groups offering support and fellowship.

Al-Anon Family Groups
61 Great Dover Street
London SE1 4YF
Tel.: 0171 403 0888 (confidential 24-hour helpline)

Support and information for families of people with alcohol problems.
AA and Al-Anon have local branches which you should be able to find in

your phone book or local services directory.

ACCEPT (Alcoholism Community for Education, Prevention, and Treatment)
724 Fulham Road
London SW6 5SE
Tel.: 0171 381 2112

ACCEPT's full name is self-explanatory.

Alcohol Concern
275 Gray's Inn Road
London WC1X 8QF
Tel.: 0171 833 3471

A campaigning and fund-raising organization that provides information and advice on treatment and services.

Turning Point
New Loom House
101 Backchurch Lane
London E1 1LU
Tel.: 0171 702 2300

Turning Point runs hostels and support services round the UK for people with alcohol, drug, and mental health problems.

Narcotics Anonymous
PO Box 1980
London N19 3LS
Tel.: 0171 240 9040

Self-help for people who want to stop and stay off drugs.

Release (National Drugs and Legal helpline)
388 Old Street
London EC1V 9LT
Tel.: 0171 603 8654 (advice line)

A charity concerned with the welfare of drug users. It offers a range of leaflets by mail order.

EATING DISORDERS

All of the following organizations offer support and counselling on eating disorders (not only anorexia nervosa):

Eating Disorders Association
Sackville Place
44 Magdalen Street
Norwich
Norfolk NR3 1JE
Tel.: 01603 621414

Anorexic Aid
The Priory Centre
11 Priory Road
High Wycombe
Buckinghamshire HP13 6SL
Tel.: 01494 21431

Women's Therapy Centre
6 Manor Gardens
London N7 6LA
Tel.: 0171 263 6200

Overeaters Anonymous
PO Box 19
Stretford
Manchester M32 9EB

SUICIDE

The Samaritans
Head office
10 The Grove
Slough
Berkshire SL1 1QP
Tel.: 01753 532713

Emergency support for people who feel lonely, desperate, or suicidal. Local branches are detailed in phone directories and local services' guides.

Compassionate Friends
See Bereavement section of this directory

CIVIL RIGHTS AND LEGAL ADVICE

The following organizations provide information specifically on mental health law:

Mental Health Act Commission
Maid Marian House
56 Hounds Gate
Nottingham NG3 6BG
Tel.: 0115 9504040

Mental Health Commission for Northern Ireland
Elizabeth House
118 Holywood Road
Belfast BT4 1NY

Mental Welfare Commission for Scotland
25 Drumsheugh Gardens
Edinburgh EH3 7RN
Tel.: 0131 225 7034

Court of Protection
The Public Trust Office Protection Division
Stewart House
24 Kingsway
London WC2B 6JX
Tel.: 0171 269 7358

The court can advise on how to deal with the estates of people (most commonly the elderly) incapacitated by mental illness. Applications to the court must be made in writing or in person.

The following organizations offer advice on a wide range of legal and civil rights issues:

The Law Society
113 Chancery Lane
London WC2A 1PL
Tel.: 0171 242 1222

The Law Society of Scotland
26 Drumsheugh Gardens
Edinburgh EH3 7YR
Tel.: 0131 226 7411

Liberty (National Council for Civil Liberties)
21 Tabard Street
London SE1 4LA
Tel.: 0171 403 3888

Notes

INTRODUCTION

1 Elizabeth Forsythe, *Alzheimer's Disease: The Long Bereavement*, Faber and Faber, London, 1990, p. 44.
2 Mary Moate and David Enoch, *Schizophrenia: Voices in the Dark*, Kingsway Publications, Eastbourne, 1990, p. 49.
3 Thomas Szasz, *The Myth of Mental Illness*, Paladin/ HarperCollins, 1972, p. 13.
4 Dr Anthony Storr, *The Art of Psychotherapy*, Heinemann Medical Books, Oxford, 5th reprint 1989.
5 Derek Gale, *What is Psychotherapy?*, Gale Centre Publications, Loughton, Essex, 1989.
6 Andrews G., 'The Essential Psychotherapies', *British Journal of Psychiatry*, 162 (1993), pp. 447–51.
7 Margison F. and McGrath G., 'An Eysenck for the 1990s?' *British Journal of Psychiatry*, 163 (1993), pp. 124–5.
8 Dean C. and Gadd E. M., 'Home Treatment for Acute Psychiatric Illness', *British Medical Journal*, 301 (1990), pp. 1021–3.
9 Ed. Groves T., *Countdown to Community Care*, BMJ Publishing Group, 1993.

CHAPTER 1

1 Dale Carnegie, *How to Stop Worrying and Start Living*, Simon & Schuster, New York, 1975, p.xiii.
2 Holmes T. H. and Rahe R. H., 'The Social Readjustment Scale', *Journal of Psychosomatic Research*, 11 (1967), pp. 213–18.
3 S. Woodward and R. Lacey, *That's Life! Survey on Tranquillizers*, BBC Books, London, 1985.
4 Shirley Trickett, *Coming Off Tranquillizers and Sleeping Tablets*, Thorsons, London, 2nd edition 1991.
5 Thornicroft G. and colleagues, 'An Inpatient Behavioural Psychotherapy Unit', *British Journal of Psychiatry*, 158 (1991), pp. 362–7.
6 Goldberg D. and colleagues, *Psychiatry in Medical Practice*, Routledge, London, 1987.
7 Gelder M., Gath D., Mayou R., *Oxford Textbook of Psychiatry*, Oxford University Press, Oxford, 1985.
8 Idem.
9 Derek Llewellyn-Jones, *Everywoman: A Gynaecological Guide for Life*, Faber and Faber, 5th edition 1990 and *Everyman*, Oxford Paperbacks, 3rd edition 1991.
10 Kingsley Amis, *Jake's Thing*,

Penguin Books, London, 1980, p. 59.

11 Slater E. and Glithero E., 'A Follow Up of Patients Diagnosed as Suffering from Hysteria', *Journal of Psychosomatic Research*, 9 (1965), pp. 9–13.

12 Davidson J. R. T., 'Drug Therapy of Post-Traumatic Stress Disorder', *British Journal of Psychiatry*, 160 (1992), pp. 309–14.

13 Vaughan K. and Tarrier N., 'The Use of Image Habituation Training with Post-Traumatic Stress Disorders', *British Journal of Psychiatry*, 161 (1992), pp. 658–64.

CHAPTER 2

1 Shirley Trickett, *Coping with Anxiety and Depression*, Sheldon Press, London, 1989, p. 41.

2 Brown G. W., Harris T. O., *Social Origins of Depression: A Study in Women in London*, Tavistock Publications, London, 1978.

3 Such as Palmer R. L. *et al*, 'Childhood Sexual Experiences with Adults Reported by Female Psychiatric Patients', *British Journal of Psychiatry*, (160) 1992, pp. 261–5.

4 Harris B., Lovett L., Newcombe R. G. *et al*, 'Maternity Blues and Major Endocrine Changes: Cardiff Puerperal Mood and Hormone Study II', *British Medical Journal*, 308 (1994), pp. 949–53.

5 Jane Price, *Motherhood: What It Does to Your Mind*, Pandora Press, London, 1988, p. 16.

6 Idem, p. 125.

7 Gath D. and Iles S., 'Depression and the Menopause', *British Medical Journal*, 300 (1990), pp. 1287–8.

8 Ballinger C. B., 'Psychiatric Aspects of the Menopause', *British Journal of Psychiatry*, 156 (1990), pp. 773–87.

9 Pamela Ashurst and Zaida Hall, *Understanding Women in Distress*, Tavistock/Routledge, London, 1989.

10 P. K. Thomas, 'The Chronic Fatigue Syndrome: What Do We Know?', *British Medical Journal*, 306 (1993), pp. 1557–8.

11 Eccleston D., 'The Economic Evaluation of Antidepressant Drug Therapy', *British Journal of Psychiatry*, 163 (1993), suppl. 20 pp. 5–6.

12 Ken Kesey, *One Flew Over the Cuckoo's Nest*, Picador/Pan Books, London, 1973, p. 146.

13 Rogers A., Pilgrim D., and Lacey R., *Experiencing Psychiatry: Users' Views of Services*, Macmillan, London, 1993.

14 Moran Campbell, *Not always on the Level*, BMJ Publishing Group, London, 1988, pp. 241–2.

15 O'Connell R. A. and colleagues, 'Outcome of Bipolar Disorder on Long-term Treatment with Lithium', *British Journal of Psychiatry*, 1991.

CHAPTER 3

1 Mary Moate and David Enoch, op. cit., pp. 61–2.

2 Dylan Thomas, *Under Milk Wood*, J. M. Dent & Sons Ltd,

London, 1977 (Everyman Paperback edition 1982, p. 60).

3 Thomas C. S. and colleagues, 'Psychiatric Morbidity and Compulsory Admission among UK-born Europeans, Afro-Caribbeans, and Asians in Central Manchester', *British Journal of Psychiatry*, 163 (1993), pp. 91–9.

4 O'Callaghan E. O. and colleagues, 'Risk of Schizophrenia in Adults Born After Obstetric Complications and Their Association with Early Onset of Illness: A Controlled Study', *British Medical Journal*, 305 (1993), pp. 1256–9.

5 Sham P. C. and colleagues, 'Schizophrenia Following Prenatal Exposure to Influenza Epidemics Between 1939 and 1960', *British Journal of Psychiatry*, 13 (1992), pp. 320–8.

6 Crow T. and colleagues, 'Schizophrenia and Influenza' *Lancet* 338 (1991), pp. 116–17.

7 R. D. Laing and Aaron Esterson, *Sanity, Madness and the Family*, Tavistock Publications, London, second edition 1984, pp. 11–12.

8 Thomas S. Szasz, op. cit., p. 17.

9 Romme M. A. J., Honig A., Noorthoorn E. O., and colleagues, 'Coping with Hearing Voices: An Emancipatory Approach', *British Journal of Psychiatry*, 161 (1992), pp. 99–103.

CHAPTER 4

1 Simone de Beauvoir (translated by Patrick O'Brian), *Old Age*, Penguin Books, London, 1977 (first published by Editions Gallimard as *La Vieillesse*, 1970), p. 10 of introduction to 1988 reprint.

2 Elizabeth Forsythe, op. cit., p. 11.

3 O'Connor D. W. and colleagues, 'Problems Reported by Relatives in a Community Study of Dementia', *British Journal of Psychiatry*, 156 (1990), pp. 835–41.

4 Deary I. J. and Whalley L. J., 'Recent Research on the Causes of Alzheimer's Disease', *British Medical Journal*, 297 (1988), pp. 807–10.

5 Harrison P., 'Alzheimer's Disease and Chromosome 14. Different Gene, Same Process?', *British Journal of Psychiatry*, 163 (1993), pp. 2–5.

6 Corder E. and colleagues, 'Gene Dose of Apolipoprotein E Type 4 Allele and the Risk of Alzheimer's Disease in Late Onset Families', *Science*, 261 (1993), pp. 921–23.

7 Eagger S. and colleagues, 'Tacrine in Alzheimer's Disease', *British Journal of Psychiatry*, 160 (1992), pp. 36–40.

8 Mowadat H. R. and colleagues, 'Sporadic Pick's Disease in a 28-year-old Woman', *British Journal of Psychiatry*, 162 (1993), pp. 259–62.

CHAPTER 5

1 Aldous Huxley, *Brave New World*, Chatto & Windus, 1977 edition (Triad/Panther edition 1977, p. 127).

2 *Mental Illness: The Fundamental*

Facts, Mental Health Foundation, 1993.

3 Neustatter Angela, 'Parental Agony and the Ecstasy', *Independent on Sunday*, 11 April 1993, p. 65.

4 Marshall E. J. and Murray R., 'The Familial Transmission of Alcoholism', *British Medical Journal*, 303 (1991), pp. 72–3.

5 Neustatter A., op. cit.

6 Ewing J. A., 'Detecting Alcoholism: The CAGE Questionnaire', *Journal of the American Medical Association*, 252 (1984), pp. 1905–7.

7 Marmot M. and Brunner E., 'Alcohol and Cardiovascular Disease: The Status of the U-shaped Curve', *British Medical Journal*, 303 (1991), pp. 565–8.

8 Ed. Paton A., 'ABC of Alcohol', *British Medical Journal*, 1988.

9 Velleman R. and Orford J., 'The Adult Adjustment of Offspring of Parents with Drinking Problems', *British Journal of Psychiatry*, 162 (1993), pp. 503–16.

10 Edwards G. and colleagues, 'Alcoholism: A Controlled Trial of Treatment and Advice', *Journal of Studies on Alcohol*, 38 (1977), pp. 1004–31.

11 Gossop M. and colleagues. 'Opiate Withdrawal: Inpatient v Outpatient Programmes . . .', *British Medical Journal*, 293 (1986), pp. 103–4.

12 See Jansen K. L. R., 'Non-medical Use of Ketamine', *British Medical Journal*, 306 (1993), pp. 601–2.

13 Mott J., 'Self-reported Cannabis Use in Great Britain in 1981', *British Journal of Addiction*, 80 (1985), pp. 37–43.

14 Thornicroft G., 'Cannabis and Psychosis: Is There Epidemiological Evidence for Association?', *British Journal of Psychiatry*, 157 (1990), pp. 25–34.

15 Neustatter A., op. cit.

16 Ron M. A., 'Volatile Substance Abuse: A Review of Possible Long-term Neurological, Intellectual, and Psychiatric Sequelae', *British Journal of Psychiatry*, 148 (1986), pp. 235–46.

17 Campbell I. A., 'Nicotine Patches in General Practice', *British Medical Journal*, 306 (1993), pp. 1284–5.

18 Dr John Strang, *The Health of the Nation: The BMJ View*, BMJ Publishing Group, 1991.

19 Neustatter A., op. cit.

CHAPTER 6

1 Duchess of Windsor quoted in Susan Sontag, *Illness as Metaphor*, Penguin, London, 1990.

2 D. M. Garner, 'Pathogenesis of Anorexia Nervosa', *Lancet*, 341 (1993), pp. 1631–5.

3 Vollrath M. and colleagues, 'Binge Eating and Concerns Among Young Adults: Results from the Zurich Cohort Study', *British Journal of Psychiatry*, 160 (1992), pp. 498–503.

4 'No One Knows I Have Bulimia. It Doesn't Show', *Good Housekeeping*, August 1992, p. 56.

5 Waller G., 'Sexual Abuse as a Factor in Eating Disorders', *British Journal of Psychiatry*, 159 (1991), pp. 664–71.

6 Orbach S., *Fat is a Feminist Issue*, Hamlyn Paperbacks, 1978.

CHAPTER 7

1 Tyrer P. and colleagues, 'Personality Disorder in Perspective', *British Journal of Psychiatry*, 159 (1991), pp. 463–71.
2 Lewis G., Appleby L., 'Personality Disorder: The Patients Psychiatrists Dislike', *British Journal of Psychiatry*, 153 (1988), pp. 44–9.
3 McGuffin P. and Thapar A., 'The Genetics of Personality Disorder', *British Journal of Psychiatry*, 160 (1992), pp. 12–23.
4 Gelder M. and colleagues, *Oxford Textbook of Psychiatry*, Oxford Medical Publications, Oxford, 1985.
5 Mersky H., 'The Manufacture of Multiple Personalities', *British Journal of Psychiatry*, 160 (1992), pp. 327–40.

CHAPTER 8

1 Pritchard C., 'Is there a Link Between Suicide in Young Men and Unemployment? A Comparison of the UK with Other EC Countries', *British Journal of Psychiatry*, 160 (1992), pp. 750–56.
2 Muldoon M. F. and colleagues, 'Lowering Cholesterol Concentrations and Mortality: A Quantitative Review of Primary Prevention Trials', *British Medical Journal*, 301 (1990), pp. 309–14.
3 Colette, *Gigi*, Penguin Books, 1958.
4 Cameron I., 'Deliberate Self-poisoning: The Need for a New Approach', *Health Trends*, 22 (1990), pp. 126–8.

CHAPTER 9

1 George Bernard Shaw, *The Doctor's Dilemma*, Penguin Books, London, 1946, reprinted 1955, p. 59.
2 Gunn J. and colleagues, 'Treatment Needs of Prisoners with Psychiatric Disorders', *British Medical Journal*, 303 (1991), pp. 338–41.
3 Department of Health, Home Office, 'Review of Health and Social Services for Mentally Disordered Offenders and Others Requiring Similar Services', final summary report, HMSO, London, 1992.
4 Select Committee on Health, 'Fifth Report on Community Care: Community Supervision Orders', HMSO, London, 1993.
5 Bernadt M. and colleagues, 'Patients' Access to Their Own Psychiatric Records', *British Medical Journal*, 303 (1991), p. 967.
6 Reuler J. B. and Balazs J. R., 'Portable Medical Records for the Homeless Mentally Ill', *British Medical Journal*, 303 (1991), p. 446.

INDEX

HarperCollins Paperbacks – Non-fiction